How Hearing Loss Impacts Relationships

Motivating Your Loved One

Richard Carmen, Au.D.
Doctor of Audiology

Auricle Ink Publishers • **Sedona Arizona**

Library of Congress Cataloging-in-Publication Data

Carmen, Richard.
  How hearing loss impacts relationships – motivating
your loved one / by Richard Carmen.
      p. cm.
  Includes bibliographical references and index.
  ISBN 0-9661826-3-4 (soft cover)
  1. Deafness. 2. Hearing aids. 3. Deaf—Rehabilitation.
4. Deafness—Miscellanea. I. Title.

  RF290.C374 2005
  617.8'9—dc22

                                        2004012188

First Printing
ISBN: 09661826-3-4
Cover Concept and Development by Richard Drayton

*This book is available at special discount when ordered in
bulk quantities. Contact the publisher for more information.*

Auricle Ink Publishers
P. O. Box 20607
Sedona Arizona 86341
(928) 284-0860
www.hearingproblems.com

DISCLAIMER

This book is very direct and confrontational. It requires common sense and discretion. Application of *any* ideas from this book to relationships in your life are at your own risk and not the responsibility of the author or publisher. If you have any hesitation about how to apply concepts from this material to your life, you need to seek professional psychotherapeutic counseling and guidance from a trained, licensed and knowledgeable therapist.

Contents

Introduction
Understanding Feelings

Introduction

Understanding Feelings

This book is written for the spouse, significant other, family or friend who is confronted with the frustrations, aggravations and turmoil that stem from untreated hearing loss in someone for whom they care a great deal. If you are among this group, this book is written for you. It will offer you insights necessary to understand the nature of problems you endure when living with someone with untreated hearing loss, and guide you in implementing techniques to create positive changes not only in the resistant person you love, but just possibly, in you too.

If you believe that things will get better by sitting and waiting, then you must also be waiting for the Tooth Fairy. This book is very direct and confrontational. Implementing any ideas from this book will require your utmost common sense and discretion. In the same way you cannot drive a locomotive without knowledge, you cannot jump into a loved one's life to make changes without proper preparation. In both cases you could end up with a train wreck!

I believe the most effective way to make changes is through understanding. I will not skirt the issues in order to make you feel better. I will tell you how things are based on decades of personal, clinical and research experience as well as volumes of published data that address the problem. There may be times you need to put this book down and take a break. Other times maybe you'll be compelled to read to conclusion a section that pertains exactly to what has been going on in your closest relationship. Read at your own pace but don't give up.

Most people with hearing loss choose to do nothing about it. There are about as many Americans suffering from heart disease as those with *untreated* hearing loss. Can you imagine if 80 percent of heart disease victims resisted treatment? Surely there is no greater number of Americans needlessly suffering from any other malady than that of untreated hearing loss.

Put another way, if one loses 50 percent of high frequency hearing making it difficult to clearly hear women and children only a few feet away, it's impact can be comparable to losing 50 percent of one's peripheral vision (as found in macular degeneration) making it difficult to clearly see people standing on one's side. Those with visual problems quickly seek out treatment while people with hearing loss often put up resistance. What lies behind this resistance and what you can do about it is the focus of our exploration here.

Now then, since resistance means doing nothing about it, you have probably reached a point of feeling that this has become a greater problem for you than your loved one. In fact, the problem may have even shifted from the hearing loss itself to the outright resistance.

In 2003[1] I ran a survey question past 210 convention-attending audiologists: "Which gender (if any) do you find in your practice most resists the idea of getting hearing aids?" All respondents had to dispense hearing aids in order to qualify. The choices of answers were:

- Mostly men
- About equal
- Mostly women
- No resistance observed

Over half of those surveyed (54 percent) reported *mostly men*. By contrast, only nine percent of respondents reported *mostly women*. (It was interesting to find that 34 percent reported it was *about equal.*) Strikingly, only one percent reported *no resistance observed*. This last statistic does not mean 99 percent of people who get hearing aids resist the idea. It means that 99 percent of surveyed audiologists reported that when resistance to hearing aids was present among their patients (which in itself was not measured) it was estimated to be six times more frequent in men than women.

So, if the survey is indicative of anything, it suggests that getting new hearing aids is not quite like shopping for a new car. With this information as background and to make the writing format in this book easier, I will refer to the male gender as being your loved one—the resistant one. This also makes handling gender easier in this material. Therefore, I don't have to qualify "she" and "he" or "his" and "hers."

For the record, research shows that women acclimate better to change than men, and the average American endures hearing loss seven to ten years before finally seeking help. The interim years can be absolute misery for all involved with a loved one's untreated hearing loss. This means you and the family get dragged through the turmoil with him. As you'll discover, non-treatment must no longer be an option. There is nothing to be gained by putting off treatment. In fact, as you will learn, the adverse consequences to all involved, especially to the hard-of-hearing loved one, are staggering.

I can tell you from my own clinical experience, as well as from research, that issues surrounding hearing loss are a major contributor toward family friction and unhappiness, even leading to divorce. Many such divorcees have regretted their selfish decision to do nothing to help themselves, which in turn would have saved their marriage and increased family tranquility and security.

As you read this book you'll notice many **"Facts"** and **"Keys."** Some of these can even be used as *affirmations* for you—thoughts that can empower you toward positive action. They will be highlighted as such and easy to spot. If you review the content of this book, these are points you may want to remember. However, I will tell you that you will find it far easier to read good ideas about what you should do, but more challenging to get yourself to do them.

To understand your resistant loved one, to grasp the nature of his objections, you probably need to know more about how he interacts in the world and less about hearing loss itself, although both will be covered in this book. The onset of hearing loss for most people is gradual over many years. In roughly five percent of cases the event occurs suddenly. In such cases, this situation is distinctly different from slow progression of loss and typically resistance is not an issue.

This book will focus exclusively on people who have experienced a relatively slow progression of hearing loss over many years who either refuse to seek help or have stopped their search at a point of unsuccessful treatment (tried hearing aids and they "didn't work"). <u>This material is not about loved ones with hearing loss who are making efforts toward resolution of their problem</u>. Assumptions, intimations or conclusions from this book <u>cannot be applied to those who are making an effort toward treatment except where it is specifically stated as such</u>. [For an in-depth perspective exclusively on pursuing hearing loss and hearing aids, you may want to explore the companion book to this one.[2]]

Data show that hearing loss rarely occurs as an isolated condition. More commonly, it is associated with other health-related issues such as depression, displaced anger, heart disease, stroke and so forth. Furthermore, these co-occurring health conditions are not all associated with hearing loss in the same way. That is, some are *causes*, some are *effects* of hearing loss. For instance, heart disease can be a cause of sensorineural hearing loss while depression can be an *effect*.

So, when you explore what hearing loss is all about, you'll see that sometimes it's not a condition you can so readily put a label on because of the complexities involved. The effects of hearing loss in one's life largely depend on individual needs, the people involved, their personalities and temperaments, the degree and duration of hearing loss itself, the auditory demand and expectations, and the specific nature of the relationship between you and your loved one.

This said, what we'll do in this book is put resistance in a box so we can examine it and decide what *you* will do about it. While life of course is hardly this simple, I will offer you a framework around which you can assemble the pieces to your own puzzle, make sense of them, know what to do with it and how to positively impact the life of someone you care deeply about.

You must realize you're not alone in this uphill battle. There are 28,000,000 Americans with hearing loss. Only 20 percent have sought help for themselves. Most of the remaining 22,000,000+ people with untreated hearing loss are battling themselves and their families over a condition that could otherwise be well-compensated for through use of hearing aids. With respect to any other single health condition in the U.S., if there were 22 million Americans suffering, it would be considered *pandemic* and the government would be intervening to help resolve the crisis. That not happening—it's in your lap.

If someone is <u>reluctant</u> to get his hearing tested or pursue hearing aids, this presupposes he is *hesitant*. This is not the same thing as being *resistant*. A reluctant person can often be persuaded through common sense and logic to do something about hearing loss. However, <u>resistant</u> hard-of-hearing people have far more substantial barriers that they cannot surmount alone. The subject matter in this book focuses on resistance, not reluctance.

While everyone's situation is somewhat different, there are enough commonalties among resistant hard-of-hearing people to be able to offer meaningful insights in a book like this. Much of my approach is a heavy dose of reality with a pound of "tough love," so you need to read between the lines to know how to integrate changes to best suit your needs and those of your loved one. This book might be thought of somewhat akin to "Al-Anon" (a Twelve-Step Program for co-dependent family members of people with addiction problems). There are two core features of resistant hard-of-hearing people that can also be seen in people with issues of addiction (such as eating disorders, gambling or substance abuse): they fail to acknowledge the problem ("denial") and subsequently do not take responsibility for it (resist treatment).

A question you may ask is if this reading could in any way undermine your efforts with your loved one. Again, if you think of yourself as having fundamental common sense, the answer is a resounding NO. If you're reading this book you already recognize his intentions of not doing anything about his hearing loss. You can offer your loved one this book or any other on hearing help, but if he's truly resistant, he probably won't read it, which is precisely why you're the one taking the initiative. He's not interested because he doesn't perceive there's a problem for him. Therefore, you're entitled to know what to do in his absence of taking action. By the end of this reading you'll have a better understanding of how you both feel and a far better grasp of the options available.

You as a loving spouse, partner, friend or family member already have enormous influence with respect to what actions your loved one can take. However, you probably are not aware of your own power of persuasion, both positive and negative. Very often, the pressure you exert for him to seek help is the problem. To understand how you can best approach your loved one will require a quiet mind, a resilient spirit, willpower, patience, well-defined goals that follow an organized plan, knowledge of hearing healthcare in your community and ultimately willingness to change on your part and the part of your loved one. This latter challenge will be addressed throughout this book and is our ultimate goal to achieve.

You need to be sure that your desire for compassion is not compromised by anger, resentment or hostility. It's easy to attract such feelings in life when living with an untreated hard-of-hearing person. Often, if you don't raise your voice he can't hear you. Other times you raise your voice so you're certain he'll hear you and he accuses you of yelling at him. Dozens of examples like this can fill your day. Your willingness to forgive your loved one for his negative reactions to hearing loss will create the atmosphere for change.

The love you once held for this special person can be conflicted and confused with many other ill feelings you have, purely a result of living with someone—nothing to do with hearing loss. There may be other factors influencing your relationship (such as financial pressures, misbehaving children, work stress, feelings of resentment) which may be difficult for you to separate from the effects of your loved one's hearing loss.

Key: Before you can understand the entangled emotional issues with your loved one, you must first look at your own feelings.

If this loved one is your spouse or significant other, realize that your choice of living with him (versus separation or divorce) is a strong indicator of your commitment to the relationship. With this in mind, I'm assuming you care a great deal about him and that despite seeing negative changes in him (like flexibility turned to stubbornness, concern for others shifted to selfishness), you are sincere in your desire to create positive changes.

Fundamental to exploring this topic is understanding that resistant hard-of-hearing people want to be accepted for who they are without having to change. It may not be any different with you wanting to be accepted for who you are. He may perceive that you are already accepted for who you are, but few accept who he is (hard-of-hearing). Why can't the world accept who he is without demanding he change? This alone can be the glue that holds resistance in place. "Let me be who I already am!" But the truth is that we are all "a work in progress." Humans are not as unchanging as we sometimes like to think of ourselves. The field of psychology has long recognized that even personalities change over time. Therefore, we can accept a loved one not only for who he is, but we can also accept him *for what he is becoming* (in the most positive sense—growth and self-awareness).

What has become known as the Serenity Prayer, reported by some to have been anonymously composed, but reported by others to have been penned by St. Francis, has been used for decades in Alcoholics Anonymous. It describes with clarity the importance of giving your relationship everything you have while respecting limits:

Key: "Grant me the serenity to accept the things I cannot change, courage to change the things I can and wisdom to know the difference."

Chapter 1

Establishing a Framework for Help

Chapter 1

Establishing a Framework for Help

Most people expect loved ones to manage their life in a responsible way so long as they are capable. This includes everything from brushing their own teeth to seeking medical treatment for problems as needs arise. So when a loved one neglects what you feel is an essential need, and it persists over a period of years, it is likely to trigger very specific emotions in you. If these emotions are not held in check, the way in which you go about offering your assistance may carry overtones of anger and frustration.

Scenario 1 is the manner and tone in which many hearing healthcare practitioners find themselves face to face when a relatively unwilling loved one is coerced into the office accompanied by a family member. This is the way <u>not</u> to do it.

SCENARIO 1 (during the consultation):

Hearing Healthcare Practitioner: "Now Fred, as we've just been discussing, you would do best if you were to get two hearing aids, one for each—"

Fred: "Two!...?"

Hearing Healthcare Practitioner: "Yes. You have equal loss of hearing in both ears. Two hearing aids will offer you tremendous benefits."

Fred: (pauses—thinking.)

Sally: "I'm not going to lose my voice anymore shouting to you from across the room! And you still can't hear me! And I'm tired of repeating myself constantly! I can't do this anymore."

Fred: "For the most part, I hear you fine."

Sally: "You don't. That's why we're here, Fred."

Fred: "We're here because of <u>you</u>."

Sally: "Fred, I don't have the hearing problem, you do."

Fred: "But you're the only one who seems to complain."

Sally: "You won't even go to the movies anymore because you can't hear."

Fred: "It's the way they make those movies nowadays. Nobody can hear."

Hearing Healthcare Practitioner: "Fred? Did you come in today with the hope that after testing I'd be telling you your hearing was okay?"

Fred: "Well...I...I...*(reluctantly)*...I was hoping so."

Here's the problem. Hearing loss for Fred has been something he has not had time to come to grips with, let alone consider any alternatives (such as hearing aids). Right now, he would be the worst possible candidate for hearing aids. He would find what seemed to him to be rational reasons why they did not help or why he did not need them (for you these would become his excuses). Had Fred slowly evolved into an understanding of how his hearing loss developed and what it was doing to him and loved ones, he'd have had the insights necessary to seek help. There are many variations on this common theme of coercion.

Since we are all individuals, reasons will vary from person to person. This *must be* ascertained through loving support and encouragement, not through coercion and pressure. It will require tremendous willpower and self-control on your part because the tendency is to throw your hands up and say it's not your problem. But it is your problem. Here are some inner thoughts some frustrated patients tend to express or have felt but preferred to hold inside:

- "Wake up!"
- "Don't you get it?"
- "Don't you see how dysfunctional you are by not seeking help?"
- "Don't you see what it's doing to our relation-ship?"
- "Don't you love me enough to do something about it?"
- "Don't you know that you're hiding the problem only from yourself—everyone else sees your foolishness?"
- "How selfish can you be?"
- "Why are you doing this to all of us?"

Key: One of your challenges is to understand why your loved one opposes the idea of seeking help.

Like with anything, there's a preferred way to present your views. Even ways that seem to be right or most sensitive may not always be best. Scenario 2 presents coercion as a result of outright love, but as you'll see, it isn't enough.

SCENARIO 2 (during the consultation):

Joan*:* "Doctor, I think it's important for Mom to have hearing aids, like you say. And this is my mother so I would like to pay for them."

Hilda: "Oh Joan, you know I don't get out much anymore. Most of my close friends have passed away. My only close friend at the retirement home is Martha, and she doesn't even leave her room anymore. What need do I have to hear anything?"

Hearing Healthcare Practitioner: "Hilda, it sounds to me like you've given up on life."

Hilda: "Dearie, at my age of 98, there's nothing I haven't already heard!"

Joan: "Mom! First of all, you're 89 not 98. And second of all, among others, you have twenty-three grandchildren who love and adore you, but you can't hear them."

Hearing Healthcare Practitioner: "Hilda, by not hearing them, you're isolating yourself. The isolation you feel is often attributed to hearing loss. This in turn causes or greatly contributes to depression. And this can make one feel like you just want to be alone because of the struggle to hear. It becomes a vicious cycle."

Joan: "Do you understand what the doctor is saying, Mom?"

These are the well-meant attempts of a frustrated daughter who dearly loves her mother. She knows what's best for her and wants to see her well taken care of in her waning years. But Joan cannot get out of her own way to see that she cannot coerce her mother into something her mother does not realize she needs. To Hilda, hearing aids hold no value. In fact, hearing holds no value. She's simply given up.

Create a Need

So how do you motivate a person you love to do something he or she believes is unimportant but you believe is in their best interest? You know kind persuasion didn't work. If you force the issue, you already know you'll receive equal or greater resistance in return. You cannot offer resistance in an argument when your loved one opposes the notion of seeking help. What you need to do is use his or her own challenges to persuade, inform or educate.

SCENARIO 3 (Jill offers an <u>excellent way</u> to discuss with her husband not hearing in church):

Jill: "Do you think you heard everything the pastor said this morning?"

Don: "I think so."

Jill: "Did you hear the example he gave specifically about faith?"

Don: "I didn't hear him say anything about *faith*."

Jill: "He talked about faith."

Don: "I must have missed that."

Jill: "Are you aware you asked me to repeat several things he said?"

Don: "Yes, but I didn't think I missed that much and besides, I don't think he always used the microphone."

Jill: "You're right, but even when he stood in front of the mike you still turned to me to repeat what he said."

Don: "Because he mumbled."

Jill: "I asked Ed and Gloria if they heard the sermon

this morning and they both said they heard fine. I heard him well also. And they were sitting on the other side of you. Honey, do you think it might be something more than the pastor mumbling?"

Here's one more angle on the same interaction:

Jill: "You know, honey, you missed a lot of what the pastor had to say this morning."

Don: "I don't think I missed a thing."

Jill: "You didn't know about certain aspects of the sermon when we were discussing it later. Honey, I really miss your input in these situations. . ."

Key: Stop making your loved one wrong for failing to hear something you hear.

In the above scenario with Jill and Don, hearing loss is never even mentioned. You can see how it may not be necessary to engage in conversation about it, something that can occasionally lead to arguments. It was left up to Don to figure it out. The issue or the challenge was simply presented to him. For many hard-of-hearing loved ones, when they are quietly and kindly presented with enough of these reminders, the subtle message starts to get through.

Key: If you make your loved one defensive, you fail at the very goal you seek. Invite his participation without judgment.

Nobody likes to be punished. This again brings about the instinct of defending oneself. By nature it places one more barrier between you and your loved one. In the previous scenario, Jill is supportive of her husband. She did not present herself in an accusatory way. She did not make him feel terrible for not hearing. She merely made an observation and inquiry. By her concern, she expressed how much she cared about him missing what the pastor had to say. How she described him missing a portion of the pastor's sermon was framed with care, concern and love.

Key: If you cannot change his attitude, you must change yours.

While the previous scenario is just one example, there are countless examples from your own life with your loved one. Each time, you must make the effort to support your loved one by allowing him to understand what it is he is not hearing. It is through this realization that he will eventually come to understand how much is actually being missed.

The hundreds and eventually thousands of times this happens, your loved one does not realize how much has been missed. Of course often others do, but commonly out of courtesy they don't offer a correction.

Key: The illusion that one's hearing is normal is reinforced when others do not identify "the misses."

You must point out each event that is not heard, but do so in a way that does not make your loved one wrong. This may require great restraint and rethinking your communication style, but without doing so, you are adding to the problem because you're enabling him to continue on this path of non-reality and misery. Unless *you* change, you are the other half perpetuating the problem.

If a tree falls in a forest and your husband is there alone but doesn't hear (or see) it fall, did it fall? In your husband's reality, it did not fall. His reality is based on all his senses, so if he can't see or hear something unfold, he simply lives with the illusion that it did not occur. This is perfectly logical.

Now look at these hearing challenges in your life with him. He doesn't hear the turn signal blinking so while it drives you nuts, it's not a part of his reality. He doesn't hear the siren so he doesn't pull the car to the side of the road. He likes TV loud only because he can't hear it at your comfort level. He doesn't answer you from another room not because he's trying to aggravate you, but because he may not hear you. Oh yes, he'll ask you a question from another room and expect to hear your reply because he has not come to terms with the fact that *he cannot hear from another room!* By the same token, he'll shout back, "I can't hear you!" <u>implying that it's your fault</u>! The reality of hearing loss remains so far on the fringe of this person's consciousness that it doesn't register as being part of the equation in his communication failure.

In summary, stop blaming, stop accusing and stop making him wrong for not hearing. For some spouses, this will require great restraint. You must understand with some people how important it is for you *not* to press the issue of the problem being his hearing. For many people who have not yet developed the coping skills to adequately deal with this issue, there can be a kind of psychological decompensation. That is, the realization that hearing loss is as bad as it is can result in emotional consequences of sadness, depression, irritability, instability, confusion and so forth. [For an extensive list of these emotions, skip ahead to Table 3-5.]

In order to minimize communication conflict, there are some basic rules of communication that can help. These rules are the foundation that should both precede and follow treatment for hearing loss.

Basic Rules of Communication

There are a number of rules that govern good communication. In order for you and your significant other to engage in conversation while minimizing frustrations, you and all family members must respect these rules of engagement. It's important that you recognize these rules now before we begin delving more deeply into the problem. If you are a contributor to the problems below, you can now make the proper corrections to function within a more effective communication style.

1: Help reduce background noise levels.

It is essential to control the level of noise in your communication environment. No one can be expected to hear well even with normal hearing if the television or stereo is blaring. Talking while television is on presents unnecessary challenges. Do not expect to hear well if your baby is crying (capable of blasts up to 120 dB)—sometimes painful! If your children are playing in the same room, either ask them to quiet down or move yourselves to another room.

Key: Create the most ideal listening conditions if you expect him to ideally hear.

2: Move closer - neither of you can speak to the other from another room.

With all due respect, keep in mind that you are probably a meaningful part of the problem on this point. Since it is rather inconvenient to always have to get up and move to another room just so your loved one can hear you better, it's important to do so. You cannot engage your loved one in conversation under circumstances that are not in his best hearing interest. You may break this rule daily, but you can stop it immediately.

You both tend to break it out of poor communication habits. The solution for you is simply not to ask him questions from another room or in any meaningful way carry on a remote/distant conversation. If you are strict on your own responsible end of this rule, it will force him to change his behavior and comply as well.

3: Capitalize on preferential seating.

Another aspect of controlling his better hearing world is preferential seating. This may mean not only being in the same room, but your loved one may need to sit nearest you or the person speaking.

However, if problems still arise with hearing, then you both must resolve yourselves to facing one another when each of you speaks. This does not mean getting in each other's face so close you can kiss his nose. If you can see each other's expressions, that should work. It will require some trials to find that comfort zone, but it's there to find (discussed next in more detail in Rule #4).

If you're in a restaurant, do not accept seating that places you in the middle of the hub. Spot the noisiest areas to avoid, such as near the kitchen, live music, speakers on the wall or a party of 12 talking so loud you cannot hear yourself think. Find a corner away from it all. Corners are usually ideal because of the acoustics it can afford your loved one. Padded walls, curtains, drapes and large plants make for excellent barriers and absorbers of sound. Also, if there are two or three people your loved one intends to talk to most, be sure he's seated nearest them so he doesn't have so much noise interference to deal with.

If you're at a theater, locate the speakers, typically placed two to four on each side wall, and seat yourself accordingly. Many theaters have "dead zones" where sound is either dull or cancelled out (out of phase). Taking a seat centered between the middle right and left wall speakers is often ideal.

If you're at your place of worship, you might try to take the same action as if you're at a theater, *but it may not always work.* There are several variables involved that may prevent one from hearing well:

- the size of the facility
- the distance between you and the clergyperson speaking
- the microphone system used by the facility (lavaliere versus fixed-on-the-podium, cheap microphone versus high quality, level of output preset—that is, many in the congregation may object to excessive amplification)
- the overall quality of the amplifying system used
- the distance between the clergy and his microphone

For these reasons alone, you are probably best off sitting up front. There is one other very important solution to better hearing during worship. Special wireless infrared or FM amplifying loop systems are already installed in many houses of worship. It is a wonderful way to hear very well even with a significant hearing loss. He merely uses an earphone supplied by the church that has its own built-in volume control. The same system can be used in theaters and civic auditoriums. If your local movie theater offers this option, it would be well worth the investment of a couple hundred dollars to purchase a set of such earphones. Your loved one would have his personal set and could possibly use it for movies as well as religious services, so long as the originating frequencies were compatible with your system. It would be well worth exploring. Hearing healthcare practitioners can be helpful in your guidance here. You may also want to explore this on your own through the Internet at www.hearingloop.org and other resources.

4: Communicate face to face when needed.

Once you both have made the agreement to be in the same room, now you must agree to speak face to face unless it has been adequately demonstrated that your loved one can hear by being in the same room as you. Often, just the close proximity of being in the same room resolves the loss of power in speech that occurs when you're further apart. Communicating face to face holds a key so essential in getting the message across.

Imagine receiving a communication devoid of everything other than the message itself. Imagine if you receive an email existing of one sentence: "Oh! I'm really sorry!"

It could be very difficult to interpret such a message since the speaker might have intended sarcasm, intimidation, or even profound sincerity. A message is understood best when all channels of interpretation are utilized. Here are some pointers on why it's so important to conduct conversation with your loved one only in his presence:

• VISUAL CUES allow your loved one to capitalize on his vision. In this effort, you shouldn't be engaged in conversation with a spatula in your mouth. The kids wearing a football helmet with a face guard shouldn't be asking dad questions and expecting him to hear. Light sources must also be considered. Glare and reflections make visual cues more difficult to see. Your loved one should be expected to have the light source at his back, which is at your front—not coming at him from the front.

• GESTURES often have their own language. This is another reason why you need to create a communication environment where your loved one sees you talking. Missing a word or two may not pose a problem to you, but when your loved one can see you using your arms and hands, they are sending messages too.

• POSTURE will often reveal what words alone cannot. The position of the body, how one holds the arms and shoulders can tell you what a person is feeling. Provide these cues.

• FACIAL EXPRESSIONS include the lines on your face, the squint in your eyes, the position of your mouth and the color in your face lend clarity to the words you speak. Your loved one cannot benefit from this unless you are close enough for him to see you.

• INTONATION/INFLECTION is another benefit that adds clarity to language. The emphasis on one part of a word may well be lost when conversing room to room: con'-vict versus con-vict' differ significantly in meaning. The difference in emphasis on certain words can result in an entirely different thought. Such subtleties not only can change a meaning, but distance diminishes the impact of these added communication cues.

• CONTEXT is important because if you rapidly change the topic of conversation, you could lose your communication partner in the process. Transition thoughts are important. Also, if one of you leaves the room and a new conversation starts, initial context may be impossible to establish. For example, imagine you and your spouse are watching television while the kids are on the front lawn playing touch football. The doorbell rings. You answer the door as your spouse hollers, "Who's at the door?" What you shout back is not what he hears: "The children are getting arrested!" By now he's halfway to the front door only to learn you said, "The children are taking a rest!" This kind of thing often happens among hard-of-hearing people because many conversations, like this example, occur so out of context that there is little frame of reference in which to place it. Helping him stay focused on the message, his familiarity with the topic and its context, withholding conversation until you are face to face, and integrating the many pointers presented in this section will improve communication between you.

• PROSODY is the speed at which you speak, affecting how your message is delivered and received. Speaking more slowly is typically better in circumstances relating to getting your message across. Even BREATHING is an indicator of your message and, for the most part, breathing cannot be heard as much as it can be seen and intuitively perceived.

5: Help your loved one anticipate what you will say.

If you ask your loved one a question and he doesn't hear and understand, repeating the same question using the same words does not usually solve the problem. If he misheard it once, he is likely to mishear it again.

Since the most common configuration of hearing loss is high frequency, using consonants that are high frequency pose challenges, especially the wispy consonants like: /s/, /sh/, /t/, /th/, /ch/, /p/, /k/, /h/ and /g/. Therefore, if you make the statement, "Our son is changing his guitar strings," almost every word holds the risk of being misinterpreted by someone with normal hearing in the low frequencies but impaired high frequencies, especially if you are communicating across a room.

Thus, rephrasing with improved contextual clarity, gestures, and avoiding high frequency words can make the message audible, but this task is daunting because we don't typically think in terms of what sounds or words are low or high frequency. Here is the rephrase in lower frequencies: "Donnie broke the metal wire strings on the Martin guitar."

Vowels carry the energy in the English language while consonants carry intelligibility. You cannot shout the voiceless sound /t/ as in Tom. But you can shout /i/ across a room. To give you a better idea of the relationship between vowel and consonant energy, can you read the following message leaving out all the consonants?

I _ _i_ _ _ _a_ i_ _a_ _ _o_ _o_a_.

Now can you read the same message with all consonants but leaving out all the vowels?

_ Th_nk th_t _t m_y sn_w t_d_y.

The actual message was, "I think that it may snow today." You can see that there are many more cues with consonants and conversely no useable cues with vowels alone.

Even if letters are out of sequence in written words, you can still often get the message:

It dosne't tkae mcuh for you to firgue out waht I'm trinyg to say hree.

Translated to oral conversation, the English language is highly redundant. Many words can be missed in a thought while the message still comes through. You may hear almost everything in a message but one or two words, and often, the context of the other words provides enough information to get the message: "While she was at the sink in the _____, she dropped a pot on the floor and off popped the _____ hurling out like a Frisbee." This is true so long as the most critical thoughts (words) are received.

Familiarity with the person speaking helps a hard-of-hearing person predict what might be said, which in turn helps him "hear" more accurately. Therefore, as you might expect, he will do better with you and the family than with strangers. Thus, if he is experiencing problems with you, you can expect the situation is probably worse with others.

Try to avoid rapid shifts in subject matter. It can take your loved one several moments to grasp that the subject has changed. In the meantime he might get lost. Try to use transitional thoughts.

6. Be patient, relaxed, non-accusatory and look for the humor.

Everyone misses words from time to time. You will only enrage your loved one if you complicate the problem with accusations of not hearing well. This does not solve anything. The tools that solve the problem are in your ability to convey compassion, love and guidance for him.

We have all found misheard words to be funny from time to time. Don't let that humor slip away. My wife recently asked me if I knew the best time to "plant miracles." I thought that was a touching play on words, though I didn't have the foggiest idea what she meant. My mind went off in a million directions, thinking "how" I might plant miracles, let alone "the best time." It sounded good to me! I got thinking, maybe evening time? Over a romantic dinner? But that's not what she asked. "Do you know the best time to plant *marigolds*?"

Section Summary

All these recommendations will not solve so many hearing problems that your loved one can forget pursuing hearing aids. It is to say that with or without hearing aids, these suggestions will make life much easier for you both and will initiate a process toward improved communication.

Chapter 2

Whose Problem is it?

Chapter 2

Whose Problem is it?

One day not long ago I was working after hours. My staff had gone home, my office was closed and I was alone when a patient we'll call Mrs. Thunder walked in. Her hearing aid was not working so I invited her to have a seat in the waiting room. I took her aid back to my lab for inspection. While examining it I suddenly heard a sound in the waiting room I couldn't identify. I quietly poked my head around the corner to find Mrs. Thunder in a flurry yanking fistfuls of cellophane-wrapped hard candies from the candy jar and stuffing them in her purse. If she could have heard the sound she was making, no doubt her conduct would have been different.

Upon finally coming out to the waiting room with her repaired hearing aid, I offered her some hard candies from the jar.

"Oh no thank you," she insisted. "I never touch them!"

I just smiled and assumed she had a lot of grandchildren.

The fact is that everyday sounds are not heard by most people with untreated hearing loss. To experience what your loved one goes through living with loss of hearing, purchase a set of earplugs. Many hearing care offices provide them at no charge (gun shops and drugstores also carry them for a couple dollars). Wait for a day without a busy schedule, then upon rising in the morning, insert the earplugs and wear them all day until you get back in bed. I bet you don't make it through the day without removing them at least once or altogether. Even a one-hour experience will be worth it.

It could be helpful to carry a notepad with you, but not necessary if you have a good memory and can honestly reflect back on your experience. What you want to bear in mind are all the nuances you miss. The intonation in a person's voice. A missed word. Even subtle vocalizations that are not words but carry great meaning. Take note of your level of operating in the world on this basis. The missed joy in hearing pleasurable sounds is only one small part of this equation. The frustration, embarrassment and myriad of other emotions that accompany people repeating themselves can all build toward explosive stress and tension.

While you do this only for a day, you must realize that your loved one may live much this way every day. This means missing oral communication and many other "reality-based" sounds. That is, action taken or not taken (or thoughts perceived or not perceived) based on what we hear or do not hear.

Compassion for people who do not take their share of responsibility in obtaining healthcare becomes a big challenge. While we may feel we know what's best for someone else, it's hard to know what it's like to be inside someone else's skin.

Key: Developing compassion will enable you to better understand the challenges confronting you both.

This inner vision may not always be pleasant, but it's worthy of exploration. What follows are some tools you may find helpful.

Co-Dependence

If you serve the endless and unrewarding needs of your loved one by being his ears for him, giving into his demands against your better judgment, repeating what he misses, interpreting messages, making him feel he's okay as he is without the need to seek any remedy for his hearing problem—you are in a co-dependent relationship. He depends on you to hear and understand, and you, willingly or not, have made yourself (or been coerced into) an indispensable resource for his hearing needs. You must ask yourself how willing you are to break this cycle.

There have been endless jokes about co-dependency that touch the lighter side of this troubling, dysfunctional problem. Why did the man cross the street?—To help the chicken make a decision. And then there's the woman who was denied jury duty because she insisted <u>she</u> was the guilty party.

While the Internet is a good resource for the humorous side of co-dependency, it can also be helpful in revealing the more serious problem it poses in relationships. (You can conduct a search on the Internet to explore this further.)

Hopefully, the relationship with your loved one is far more meaningful than the simplicity of what I'm going to say next, so bear with me. In terms of the essence of co-dependence in communication with your loved one, a reason your loved one may need you is for your good hearing, and one reason you may need him is that it fulfills a purpose in you that may tie in with your need to feel good about yourself. By your action in helping him hear, it can make you <u>both feel better</u>, but it will never solve the underlying problem of him <u>hearing better</u>. If you have half a heart, of course it's human nature to want to pitch in and assist somebody in need. However, in this case, as alluded to earlier, you are perpetuating the problem. In fact, it's worth restating: *you are part of the problem!* Now don't throw this book down in disgust because I'm picking on you. Examine your relationship to recognize if what I'm saying applies to you, then do something about it.

Key: If you cannot be honest with your-self about the issues, it's impossible to be honest with him.

Co-dependence has been applied to a wide variety of healthcare issues far beyond the scope of hearing loss. The concept of co-dependence really developed in an effort to understand the role of the spouse or family member in relation to the alcoholic. For our purposes, this means that the hearing spouse *enables* the hard-of-hearing spouse (that is, facilitates the problem) by interceding and covering up the problem so that everything appears to be "fine" to the outside world. The hallmark of a co-dependent is that need to look good to the world at large. Sound familiar?

Co-dependence can occur by active support, such as constantly repeating yourself and doing anything to get your loved one to hear what is missed, or by passive support, such as you not admitting he has a hearing problem. This reflects a terribly dysfunctional relationship usually based on dishonesty with yourself or your loved one. If you're reading this book, you cannot be engaged in passive support. Nevertheless, active supporters may not realize the depth of their own involvement.

Let's Just "Fix the Problem"

A typical inclination you're likely to have is to "fix the problem." This is the tendency with co-dependency. Before you can address his issues, you need to get a handle on what you're perhaps doing to contribute to the problem.

Key: You cannot fix the problem if your loved one believes there is no problem.

You cannot get your loved one to seek treatment for hearing loss based on your insistence. It can only come by his awareness of its effect *in his world*, then his taking responsibility for it. In the meantime, this sets you up for countless frustrations that seem to have little to no resolve because it continues to affect your world and he seems oblivious to it.

Right now, it's less important that you try to change his stubbornness—because the challenge is formidable until you are fully prepared—and more essential that you understand what you feel and what options are available to you. This will then open the floodgate for change.

Thus, if this is the person you chose to partner with in life, it's terribly important that you first identify your own feelings in order to know what to do about them.

Exploring Your Issues

The following questionnaire may help you gain clarity on these feelings. Answer *Yes* (Y) or *No* (N):

____ 1. Do you feel angry that your loved one is not getting help?

____ 2. Do you think you contribute to the problem by your upset?

____ 3. Does it upset you when you have to repeat yourself?

____ 4. Do you "fill in the gaps" your loved one doesn't hear?

____ 5. Do you resent filling in these gaps?

____ 6. Do you sometimes comply with your loved one's request to avoid certain social situations because of the hearing loss and as a result do you resent this?

____ 7. Do you feel your loved one is vain?

____ 8. Do you believe your loved one's self-image (vanity) is more important than his need to hear?

____ 9. Do you resent this?

____ 10. Do you think your loved one feels it is more important to maintain the illusion of hearing normally rather than taking positive action to do something about it?

____ 11. Do you find yourself arguing with your loved one over issues of not hearing?

____ 12. Do you get frustrated socially when your loved one engages in conversations that result in obvious hearing problems?

YES to any one of the above questions indicates that you certainly have something to resolve. The more *YES* answers, the more work you have ahead of you. Answering *YES* to most or all of the questions is enough to raise a red flag. You're probably in over your head, so it's a good thing you're reading this book!

One of the more common emotions you may have noted in this questionnaire was *resentment*. It is closely tied to anger and together is the most common emotion a person will experience with a hard-of-hearing loved one who does nothing about the hearing loss. First you resent the action you must take on behalf of your loved one. Then you get mad at yourself for taking that action (like continually repeating yourself). Then you express this anger directly at your loved one! In the meantime, your loved one has no idea from where this tornado came. All these incidents can silently gather within you and can eventually culminate in your own rage.

Key: Resentment puts out the flames of passion.

The early stage of co-dependence around hearing loss is merely reaching out to help your loved one hear better. This starts quite innocently, but can eventually reach a point of your own habitual self-defeating coping mechanisms. Ultimately, as a co-dependent, you try to control more and more of your loved one's hearing needs because "He may miss something" or "because you love him" and "That's what a good _____ [wife, daughter, son, spouse, friend] does." As a result, your loved one comes to depend more and more on you without developing the need to seek professional help. In fact, why should he? It's perfect the way it is.

Or is it? Have you developed a rewarding relationship with one another or have you taken each other hostage in the dance of co-dependence?

One of the downsides to co-dependent hearing help is that old resentment you can develop. Most people get tired of the effort it takes to be someone else's ears. It becomes difficult to relax and enjoy yourself if you must "listen up" during every conversation. It also becomes a strain and distraction because you lose your concentration and connection in conversation when you must continually repeat and interpret.

Some could say, "I don't mind having to do this." This certainly seems selfless and altruistic, but if your loved one can be helped through hearing aids, this is classic co-dependence. It will never solve the core problem of having your loved one hear better on his own, at family gatherings, at work, on the telephone, during leisure moments without you, and so forth. You should stop being his ears unless he either cannot be helped with hearing aids or wears hearing aids and still needs the extra hearing clarification you provide.

Conversely, you cannot live in a vacuum completely devoid of the influences of co-dependence, nor is that our goal here. That is, <u>you have to be involved</u> in your loved one's quest for better hearing, but cautious that you do not overstep your boundaries or his, making yourself <u>solely responsible</u> for him acknowledging the problem and seeking help.

Your Own Self-Realization

The single identifier of a co-dependent loved one tied to someone with hearing loss is that *need to help*. Coming to terms with your mission of helping your loved one will better enable him to finally take action. So long as you continue to help him, you are pulling out the carpet of motivation from beneath him.

***Key: If your loved one has not yet tried
hearing aids, be sure your co-dependent
behavior is not a major factor in his
resistance. Then prepare yourself for
change.***

Change of any kind is never easy. The change
we're looking for in your loved one is huge—*independent hearing*. However, to avoid a recipe for
emotional or communication disaster, it will take
consistent and predictable effort on your part. Here
are some of the ingredients required by you to help
your loved one in a transition toward awakening him
to the need for hearing aids. They parallel the basic
rules for communication previously presented and
are fundamental to the steps toward resolving his
co-dependent hearing issues. The more you and all
family members adhere to these guidelines, the more
your loved one can anticipate what to expect from
everyone. These tips will help you establish firm
boundaries within which you can help a loved one:

1. Stop repeating yourself! Explain that
you're on a "Hearing Help Quest"—one that involves
him by allowing him the opportunity to realize how
often he asks for help. Do not stop helping him. All
you need to do is preface what you repeat for him
by each time saying, *"Hearing Help!"* In a short
amount of time he will realize how often you say
this. In turn, he will come to realize how often he
depends on you. You both may even start laughing
about it. (This suggestion is only for a loved one
who *resists* the idea of getting help. Your offer of
saying "Hearing Help" might serve his needs best in
the privacy of your home.)

2. Stop raising your voice (then complaining you're hoarse). This results in stressing your throat and vocal chords.

3. Stop being the messenger by carrying the communication burden for your loved one. Do not report "He said" and "She said" when he needs to be responsible for getting this information directly from the source.

4. Do not engage in conversation from another room as tempting as this is and as convenient as it appears. This sets up your communication process for failure.

5. Create a telephone need. This means for you to stop being his interpreter on the telephone. Allow him to struggle and even fail in order to recognize how much help he needs. We're looking for motivation (to hear) from him—not you. By continuing to help him in this regard, you are depriving him of one more communication channel that he may well be able to use effectively with hearing aids (especially receiving calls on a speaker phone).

Levels of Resistance

There are many levels of resistance from which you will need to identify your loved one's level as shown in Table 2-1. This is not to suggest that your loved one will move from one level to another or that there is any sequence to these levels. There is not. However, <u>all resistant hard-of-hearing people get trapped at a point that results in inaction</u>. It's this inaction you will need to identify in Table 2-1. Once you recognize it, you will then know how to best proceed. There may even be two or three levels of resistance coexisting.

Table 2-1: Levels of resistance.

Denial
- Does not believe he has a hearing problem.
- Cannot talk about the hearing problem.

Inaction
- Complains he can't hear but seeks no treatment
- Had a hearing assessment but did not follow hearing healthcare practitioner's recommendation of getting hearing aids.

Failed Action (includes):
  - *Stubbornness*
  - *Negative Attitude*
  - *Control Issues*
  - *Passive-Aggressive Behavior*

Examples of Failed Action:
- Insisted on hearing aids not recommended and now cannot hear with them (may be *stubbornness*).
- Purchased hearing aids but he won't wear them (*stubbornness*).
- Purchased hearing aids only to prove they cannot work for him (may be a *negative attitude*).
- Purchased hearing aids, but turns them off most of the time while wearing them (may be a *control issue*).
- Purchased hearing aids but only wears them when he wants to, not when he always needs to (may be a control issue or *passive-aggressive behavior*).

Denial

- *"Does not believe he has a hearing problem."*

- *"Cannot talk about the hearing problem."*

Denial of hearing loss in the early stages of its progression is actually quite common. I remember when my waist shifted from belt size 30 to 32. I called the salesman over to ask if my favorite belt manufacturer was trying to save on leather by making shorter belts! The first thought was not the possibility that my waist was a little chunkier.

When confronted with the truth of a situation, if one persists in rebuking whatever truth confronts them, this is denial. In more clinical psychological terms, denial can be defined as a "Failure to acknowledge an unacceptable truth or emotion or to admit it into consciousness, used as a defense mechanism."[3]

When we consider the many painful experiences a hard-of-hearing person goes through with hearing loss, they might seem justified in denying the problem. After all, who would welcome such turmoil? But true denial of hearing loss occurs before the emotions have even struck. That is, if one misses hearing something, he attributes it to being the way someone said it or the circumstances of room acoustics or brushes it off as nobody can ever hear so-and-so anyway when she speaks. The notion that the problem is *his* is so repressed it doesn't register in his consciousness.

When people realize that the problem is their hearing and not the circumstances of the environment or something else, it can be alarming. Hearing healthcare practitioners inform their patients of this daily, with many patients hoping the problem is not their hearing.

Provided with this information and choosing to do nothing about it when a hearing healthcare practitioner offers help is not denial, but *resistance*. While true denial is rare among hard-of-hearing people experiencing hearing loss for years, resistance is common, as the survey pointed out at the beginning of this book. The vast majority of untreated hard-of-hearing people in the U.S. (22,000,000+ people) do not seek treatment for reasons that cannot be rationally justified (as cited in Table 2-1).

Key: The fact that treatment is not sought is denial of treatment and cannot automatically be construed as denial of the presence of hearing loss.

In the extreme case of *real denial*, you should proceed cautiously because it's the psyche's way of dealing with the problem. To confront someone in real denial could result in psychological decompensation—a disintegration of their defense mechanisms that have been protecting them. You do not want to suddenly thrust your loved one into crisis, confronting issues before he is psychologically prepared to deal with them. In such cases, psychological intervention by a licensed and trained therapist might be an option. This will be discussed in the next chapter.

The fact that your loved one may not be able to talk to *you* about his hearing problem does not preclude that he cannot talk about it or that he's in denial. He may not feel safe with you, feeling that perhaps you may have an ulterior motive (like treatment), you may berate him, or the topic brings up feelings of embarrassment, and so forth.

Under the umbrella of therapy, you can safely express your concerns in his presence without the greater risk of decompensation. It also gives the person who would like to talk about it (a non-denier) an opportunity to express his views on the matter in an environment of safety and comfort. Since getting him to agree to go to therapy in itself may pose a problem, you can do so on the grounds that it is *you* who needs to discuss issues, without being specific and leaving his issues out of it altogether. Therapy also does not necessarily presuppose long term. Sometimes only a few sessions are so valuable that it launches people into taking the action necessary.

Once in therapy, you can express you love him and want to be able to communicate better. You can reveal how his problem impacts the life of everyone in the family and that his decision not to acknowledge it or do nothing about it presents unnecessary challenges for the entire family. This open dialog will be the stepping stone upon which all future hearing aid treatment is based. If this dialog gets as far as him being willing to see a hearing healthcare practitioner, taking a hearing exam and even trying hearing aids, it would be ideal to do so under the guidance of this therapist.

Inaction

- *"Complains he can't hear but seeks no treatment."*

- *"Had a hearing assessment but did not follow hearing healthcare practitioner's recommendation of getting hearing aids."*

If your spouse or loved one complains he cannot hear but does nothing about it, there's one or more issue blocking him. You merely need to find out what that is and do something to solve it. Don't merely listen to him verbalize the problem and accept it. Some people who decline to seek treatment for hearing loss feel it is a sign of weakness or aging. Others perceive it as an indicator they are handicapped, an idea some refuse to accept. The root of the problem must be uncovered before proper action can be taken.

Key: If you want results, influence change rather than embracing inaction.

Jump ahead and take a look at Table 4-1 and note the top reasons hard-of-hearing people give for not using hearing aids. If you can nail down his true objection, you can address it. If he won't tell you, then the problem persists. The state of inaction may seem to you a place he's been teetering for years, but I assure you it can take only a small push from here to propel him forward into action. You must be persistent in your discovery of the obstacle(s) in his way and tolerant of his resistance. Kindness will go a very long way. If he knows he has your sincere support, it may be enough for him to get going.

Some resistant hard-of-hearing people go as far as the hearing assessment but shortchange themselves and their family by not getting hearing aids. Again, you must uncover his particular objections. Do not beat it out of him! If this is your spouse, you know him well. Search for explanations. Try to match your loved one's needs and demands with the most appropriate personality type of the hearing healthcare practitioner you select. Your loved one must have an open, honest relationship with a hearing healthcare practitioner he likes, trusts and is really comfortable with.

You know best how to get to the core of the issue. Go for it. Find the objection and work with him to resolve it. Inject humor and love, something often missing for years in such relationships because of the hearing loss (and overall life chal-lenges).

This may go against you personally because you may be feeling so angry for so long that contem-plating kindness or forgiveness in order to get him on his feet may seem beyond your call of duty. Think positively and optimistically. It's contagious. Your support is pivotal to the results everyone is seeking.

Failed Action

Failed action is simply a process where one has made efforts toward treatment but for whatever reasons, the end result was no hearing aids. This may have been due to any number of facts or misfortunes which include stubbornness, negative attitude, control issues or passive-aggressive behavior. It could also have been due to problems in the hearing aid fitting, the wrong time to proceed due to other problems, financial considerations and so forth.

Here are some common experiences of hard-of-hearing people who went as far as getting hearing aids, but failed in their use. See if you recognize familiarity with any of these as they relate to your loved one (from Table 2-1):

- Insisted on hearing aids not recommended and now cannot hear with them (may be stubbornness).
- Purchased hearing aids but he won't wear them (may be stubbornness).
- Took the hearing test and made purchase of hearing aids only to prove they cannot work for him (can be a negative attitude).
- Purchased hearing aids, but turns them off most of the time while wearing them (may be a control issue).
- Purchased hearing aids but only wears them when he wants to, not when he always needs to (may be a control issue or passive-aggressive behavior).

Stubbornness

If you are dealing with failed action, he is the closest of all levels to getting help. It may not seem so living with his state of mind, but a small bump can get him back on track. Failed action is sometimes better than no action at all. In fact, the average American waits seven to ten years before taking the positive action of getting hearing aids. You are not likely to be spending that kind of time in failed action. If something goes wrong, it can be rectified.

If your loved one received hearing aids that he wanted, but not the ones recommended by the hearing healthcare practitioner, it usually comes down to either a financial or cosmetic issue, more often the latter. In the 1990s, hearing industry manufacturers developed the smallest hearing aid ever (completely-in-the-canal: CIC). They were at the time the most expensive hearing aids on the market but wearers didn't care. People were gladly willing to pay the extra money so the hearing aids couldn't be seen.

The downside to this breakthrough in miniaturization was that many people who should not have been wearing them began ordering them. It was not possible to install a power circuit into a tiny shell, so lots of hard-of-hearing people were not hearing well, but they looked great because no one could see the hearing aids. This problem persists even today.

You'll know your spouse or loved one *has arrived* when you hear him say, "I don't care what they look like, I want to hear better!" It's not uncommon in practice to find a patient wearing CIC hearing aids who suddenly accepts behind-the-ear instruments and is flabbergasted at not only the quality of sound, but what he has been missing because of his issues around vanity. Hearing healthcare practitioners are trained to know what will sound best for their patients.

Negative Attitude

I would be lying if I said that a hearing aid trial is a piece of cake for everybody. It is for some and not for others. It requires a positive attitude. Some frustrations can be expected. This is a whole new experience, but some people let little frustrations get in the way. This is where your support will be critical. Maintain a sense of humor. This is not the end of the world.

No matter the problem, if your loved one is frustrated with something around the hearing aid experience, get back with your hearing healthcare practitioner. Work as quickly as you can to address whatever problems arise in order to avoid unnecessary delays and frustrations. Do not wait for things to get better on their own. They sometimes don't and it's not worth the risk. In the worst case scenario, your loved one may simply throw the hearing aids in a drawer. One bad moment for some people can make the entire experience negative. This is one of the most important roles for the family. The hearing healthcare practitioner will welcome your loved one back so the problem can be solved.

Some people who are pushed into hearing aids too soon in their unresolved resistance end up rejecting them. They will use any excuse to justify that these things just aren't for them. This is why it's so important to have a good sense of timing and respect for your loved one's readiness.

Control Issues

If your spouse purchased hearing aids, but either wears them *only when he wants to*, not when he *needs to*, or turns the volume off most of the time while still wearing them, this is indicative of control issues. This is purposeful behavior (unlike passive-aggressive acts), perhaps even an attempt at feeling he still has control of his world.

Some hearing aids of the past (typically analog) could not regulate sound. With the advent of 100 percent digital hearing instruments, most have become self-regulating (loud sounds are softened, soft sounds are made louder). Thus, if your loved one finds that he can hear television well without hearing aids (maybe he's using an amplified earphone set), can talk on the telephone with no problems (maybe he has a built-in amplifier), then maybe he only needs the hearing aids for specific situations. Therefore, he innocently turns them off or removes them.

On the other hand, if you notice he's not wearing them, cannot hear you and this is a repeated pattern, there's a problem. This brings us to the next more serious issue.

Passive-Aggressive Behavior

Passive-aggressive behavior occurs by *subconscious sabotage of another person* and is seen often in couples. This behavior does not occur occasionally or by accident. For example, patients of mine George and Esther were watching television together in the living room with a bowl of peanut brittle between them when Esther dozed off. She had removed her small in-the-canal hearing aids prior to dozing but did not realize she plopped them right into the bowl. George, eager for more peanut brittle ended up chewing both of her hearing aids to pieces. A true story, but not one of passive-aggressive behavior, as this was an accident.

An example of passive-aggressive behavior is telling your spouse that you're going out with friends later on and to please remember to wear his hearing aids so he can be part of the conversation. You get to the restaurant and he's forgotten the hearing aids. Bet this has happened a few times in your life if your loved one owns hearing aids!

If your spouse wears hearing aids, passive-aggressive behavior gets real murky because this can be a two-way street. For example, *you* make plans to go out to dinner with another couple. *You* make the reservations at a new trendy restaurant that is very noisy and hard to hear. Your spouse remembers to wear his hearing aids but is overcome by the background noise and is left out of most conversation for the evening. In this case, you sabotaged your husband.

Passive aggression is covert behavior that on the surface does not appear to be what it is. It can be displayed as stubbornness, but is also characterized by procrastination, obstruction and inefficiency. On the surface it masks itself as kindness or cooperation when in fact there is deep, underlying hostility. Such a person is resistant to getting help that will result in an end to the problem. There may be a million excuses or you may even get a commitment, even a date, but it never happens. Worse, despite the fact that your loved one depends on you, he finds fault with you. This slowly builds your own hostilities and resentments.

This covert way of expressing hostility is found commonly among couples quite apart from hearing loss. This learned behavior style centers around and leads to lack of intimacy. It is not a healthy way to coexist or manage relationships and it can be surmounted. Coming up shortly are 10 steps to *independent hearing*. This will help you put a handle on this problem If you sense it characterizes your relationship—on one or both sides.

Who Owns the Hearing Loss?

This book assumes you already know your loved one has a hearing problem and for all intents and purposes he knows it. You just need to find a way to gently nudge him to do something about it. He cannot do something about it until he literally "owns" it, takes possession of it, holds responsibility for the problem.

One of the easiest things you no doubt already have tried is to get him seen for a hearing assessment with a hearing healthcare practitioner. I suspect that if this had been your easiest option, you'd have done it already and you wouldn't be reading this book. In order for you not to be a co-dependent partner, the appointment-making must originate from the hard-of-hearing spouse. This demonstrates that *he* owns his hearing loss, not *you*.

Another effort toward him owning the problem is for him to take a hearing screening questionnaire (one is provided in Table 2-2). If he has been extremely resistant to hearing help, this may be a relatively safe and harmless way for him to begin to recognize that there is a problem. However, the manner in which you present the invitation for him to take it will be crucial to his receptivity to actually taking it.

If you throw this in front of him, you are ensnared into co-dependency again. While you cannot operate totally devoid of interaction with him if you are to help him, you must choose your inter-actions carefully, minimizing (but not necessarily eliminating) co-dependent behaviors.

You cannot approach your loved one with the intention of proving that he has a hearing loss even if you think it's in his best interest. You need to find a way that either makes this fun or informative for him. Perhaps this could be a family hearing screening that everybody takes, including the kids. So long as the focus is off of him (if this is an issue) he might be more receptive.

This is not intended as a *diagnostic procedure*, but rather for general inquiry and hopefully discus-sion.

If you or your loved one answered YES to even one question in Table 2-2, there may be a problem. If any three questions were YES, this only confirms what you already suspect or know. He has a hearing problem. This strongly suggests that he needs to be

Table 2-2: Hearing Screening

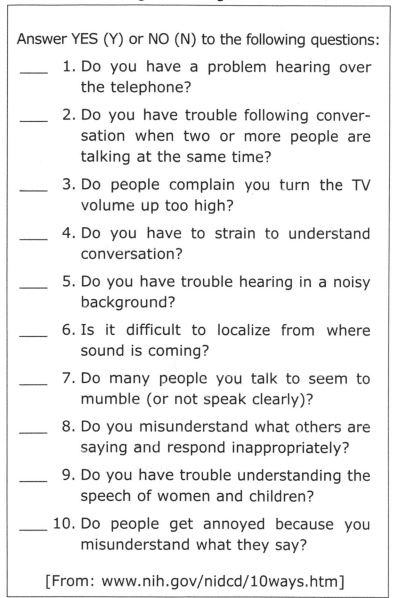

Answer YES (Y) or NO (N) to the following questions:

____ 1. Do you have a problem hearing over the telephone?

____ 2. Do you have trouble following conversation when two or more people are talking at the same time?

____ 3. Do people complain you turn the TV volume up too high?

____ 4. Do you have to strain to understand conversation?

____ 5. Do you have trouble hearing in a noisy background?

____ 6. Is it difficult to localize from where sound is coming?

____ 7. Do many people you talk to seem to mumble (or not speak clearly)?

____ 8. Do you misunderstand what others are saying and respond inappropriately?

____ 9. Do you have trouble understanding the speech of women and children?

____ 10. Do people get annoyed because you misunderstand what they say?

[From: www.nih.gov/nidcd/10ways.htm]

seen by an **Audiologist** (whose practice centers around the assessment and rehabilitation of people with hearing loss, including prescribing appropriate hearing aids), a **Hearing Instrument Specialist** (whose practice centers around the actual dispensing of hearing aids), or by an **Otologist** (a medical practitioner whose practice centers around diagnosis and medical treatment of hearing loss).

It is possible that your loved one's hearing problem can be very simply resolved. It could be a slow but progressive accumulation of earwax or a chronic middle ear infection due to a build-up of fluid. Both can be medically addressed, successfully treated and fully resolved with no residual hearing loss remaining. However, without an assessment, it becomes impossible to determine the problem.

Something seemingly as benign as earwax can fester and lead to infections and a wide variety of bacterial or fungal growth in the ear canal (such as salmonella). Infectious middle ear fluids that are not treated can lead to permanent sensorineural hearing loss.

If you were successful in getting your loved one to take the hearing screening and it indicated a possible hearing problem, the next step is to make the leap to a more reliable assessment by a hearing healthcare practitioner. If he still resists, he needs to know the potentially serious consequences of his neglect (discussed at length in the next chapter). The old notion that *discretion is the better part of valor* never held truer than now. Let knowledge, common sense and your own intuitive feelings guide you.

10 Steps to Your Loved One's "Independent Hearing"

Now that you have a better understanding of co-dependence, it's time to address *independence*. There are 10 easy steps to help you resolve the dilemma of co-dependency by recognizing the simple and practical guidelines for your loved one's *independent hearing*. These steps basically unravel your co-dependency. While the following can apply to both of you, you cannot snag him into this as long as he remains resistant to help. Therefore, these points apply only <u>to you</u> for the time being:

1. Stop supporting a system of communication that does not work.
2. Set new boundaries by changing your priority in communication from *needing to help him hear* to *only managing your own communication needs*.
3. Accept the probability that he will fail in communication and that's okay because it's part of a process toward treatment.
4. If you do not remain his ears, he may find someone else to lean on. That's okay. Just don't make him wrong for it.
5. Trust yourself, maintaining your own high self-esteem without having to fall back into a cycle of hearing for him just because he expects it.
6. Control your fear—you cannot use your own *fear of conflict with him* as an excuse to avoid making changes that will benefit you both (because *you already have conflict!)*
7. Be truthful with yourself AND start being truthful with him on how his hearing problem impacts you, speaking from your heart, not from anger.
8. Give him choices, options and helpful alternatives, but do not give him demands, threats and consequences.
9. Find in this book just <u>one</u> sensitive way to broach the topic of him seeking treatment.
10. Accept no excuses, but realize that no matter what you do he may not change and it's not your fault.

Chapter 3

Consequences of
Untreated Hearing Loss

Chapter 3

Consequences of Untreated Hearing Loss

It is worth repeating: untreated hearing loss comprises the vast majority of the estimated 28,000,000 Americans with hearing loss: more than 22,000,000 Americans have not taken action to help themselves.

Fact: There now is scientific evidence that shows untreated sensorineural hearing loss can result in a variety of other health-related problems.

Depression

A common condition found among co-dependent relationships is depression. More than 18,000,000 people age 18 and older have a diagnosable depressive disorder in the U.S.[4] The disease burden of mental illness on health and productivity in the U.S. is more than the disease burden caused by all cancers.[5] The average age of onset is the mid-20s, it affects twice as many women as men, and by the year 2020, it is projected that mental illness will increase its present burden on society by 50 percent.[6] Typically, depression associated with hearing loss happens gradually as the hearing loss becomes more debilitating.

If you've been trying to sway your loved one toward seeking hearing help, but are met with persistent resistance, it is possible that depression could be an underlying cause. Ideally, it might be highly informative for you (and your loved one) to complete the simple questionnaire in Table 3-1. It shows the symptoms of depression in older adults.

If a YES response occurs to four or more of these symptoms and the symptoms have been present for two weeks or longer, depression may be a factor. A psychological evaluation and/or treatment may be indicated. At this point, consulting your physician or licensed therapist would be an advisable next step.

Hearing Loss and Depression are Corroborated

The presence of hearing loss in and of itself may be a contributor to depression. A study by Bridges and Bentler[7] revealed that depression was significantly more prevalent among those with hearing loss. In a six-year longitudinal study by Wallhagen and his team[8] which comprised 356 hard-of-hearing men and women age 65 and older, there was more than a three-fold likelihood of depression at the six-year follow-up among the hard-of-hearing participants.

In yet another study comprising over two thousand subjects,[9] researchers concluded that participants reporting moderate or more hearing impairment were twice as likely to be depressed as persons reporting no hearing loss.

This should be eye-opening news. But just as intriguing is a study reported by Sergei Kochkin, Ph.D. (Executive Director of the Better Hearing Institute) and Carole M. Rogin, M.A (Executive Director of the Hearing Industries Association) in

Table 3-1: Symptoms of Depression in Older Adults.[10-11] Check those that apply to you and your loved one. [www.nimh.nih.gov/publicat/over65.cfm]

Your-Self	*Loved One*	*Depressive Symptoms*
____	____	very tired, slowed down, fatigued
____	____	in a persistently sad mood
____	____	a change in behavior, e.g., overall withdrawal from social support, unopened mail.
____	____	not enjoying things the way I used to
____	____	restless or irritable
____	____	difficulty concentrating
____	____	sleeping more or less than usual
____	____	eating more or less than usual
____	____	persistent headaches, stom-achaches, or chronic pain
____	____	nervous or empty
____	____	guilty, worthless or helpless
____	____	hopeless
____	____	life is not worth living
____	____	no one loves me
____	____	an absence of pleasures or joy
____	____	excessive crying

conjunction with the National Council on Aging and Market Research, Inc.[12-13] They found that family members consistently reported more depression in their loved ones than patients themselves admitted. Thus, you can be a very important team player in the restoration of hearing health in your loved one.

If he suffers from one or more other chronic health conditions such as cancer, cardiovascular disease, neurological disorders, various metabolic disturbances, arthritis and sensory loss, research shows there is a greater probability that he will be depressed.[14]

You need to bear in mind that while *hopelessness* and *social isolation* are two red flag effects of hearing loss, they both are larger indicators of depression. They are intricately interwoven. The presence of hearing loss that leads to social embarrassment can eventually diminish the joy of being with people. Such isolation can then lead to depression.

The reason you need to be concerned about other health-related conditions is that research[11] has shown that depression occurs in 25 percent of individuals undergoing medical treatment, and that about half of all medical patients do not comply with treatment recommendations. This will directly impact your quest for better hearing health in the one you love. He cannot succeed at hearing health until his depression has been addressed. To do otherwise may risk an unpleasant experience. Your loved one should be prepared to function socially, and while you expect success with new hearing aids, if depression is undetected or untreated, you're leading with the best intentions but the wrong foot forward.

I do offer one caution to you. Your loved one's

depression may be related to issues other than hearing loss (vis-à-vis his marriage, children, employment, and so forth). It's not even necessary for you to identify causality so long as you inspire your loved one to seek psychotherapeutic help if you suspect the presence of depression. Let professionals do the assessment.

Interventions

If there is hearing aid resistance on your loved one's part along with depression, it may take gentle family encouragement or even *psychological intervention*. If you conduct such an intervention, this is a very specific and psychologically based approach that can pull a loved one out of their state of mind. It has been used for years with alcoholics unable to break the addiction. This is not something to attempt alone but with the family and a trained therapist. Keep in mind that true denial, that is absolute denial of the existence of hearing loss, is far beyond the scope of what any family can address without expert counsel. Families are not equipped for the consequences of such confrontation.

The goal of intervention is to get your loved one to confront the behavior he cannot change (whether it's substance abuse, physical abuse, survivorship, posttraumatic stress, etc). While hearing loss may seem to be a stretch as a basis for intervention, if your loved one is truly in denial, the challenge is as real as if you were dealing with any addiction or trauma. If issues of a true denier affect every member of the family and the loved one refuses all help, a family may have no choice but to create an intervention, especially if a loved one's hearing loss progresses and close relationships suffer.

Intervention occurs with no advance warning and at a predetermined time and place. This is commonly done in the home at a time he may be most receptive (like on a Saturday afternoon), avoiding times he may be more stressed (such as after a long work day).

It is essential for the sake of impact that all family members attend (spouse and children). This is the beginning of his support network that will see him through. Often, the resistant person is surprised that everyone feels so strongly about his hearing loss. He may feel very moved that he is loved and cared enough about for everyone to come together in this way, or he may resent it deeply. This is why psychotherapeutic guidance is so important.

Everyone gets to present how they feel and how they have been affected. This is expressed in loving terms with a focus on the positive and hopeful. It is a useful tool for change in the most highly resistant behaviors. But it can also be effective as a one-time event.

Since exceptionally few people with hearing loss function at a level of true denial, in situations where you and perhaps the family find yourself able to talk with your loved one about his barriers to getting help, he would likely be a good candidate for a "family discussion" or "outing" without a therapist. This holds the same function as an intervention. This can be a powerful event in your loved one's life and can often create a pivotal shift from *inaction* to *action*. It boils down to love and communication.

What follows are snippets from a transcript of a psychotherapeutic intervention in a therapist's office with Sue, two teenage kids and Tim the resistant husband with untreated hearing loss who declined hearing aid use.

Therapist: "Tim, as you know, Sue has been coming here for five months on her own and we've had a chance to discuss many issues, some of it being her depression. Today your whole family has come in to talk about an issue that is troubling the family. Each of your family members would like to talk to you about how your hearing loss has impacted them."

Tim: "I don't see my hearing loss as an issue!"

Therapist: "I respect that that's how you feel, but nonetheless, your family has something to say."

Tim: "Everyone else is bothered but me. I do fine!"

Billy: "Dad, my experience is that there are many things I say to you that you don't hear. I really want to be able to have conversations with you. I love you very much and you not addressing this problem is painful to me."

Tim: "Painful? How?"

Billy: "I feel I don't have as much of a relationship with you as I could because communication is such a struggle."

Tim: "Billy, when my mind is on things I'm not a good listener."

Therapist: "Tim, may I suggest you allow everyone here to say what they need to say without you feeling you need to respond."

Renee: "Dad, there are so many times I need your advice and help but I feel like I can't turn to you because when I talk with you, you don't always hear what I say. I miss being able to have the talks we used to have. I love you and want you to do something about your hearing."

Sue: "Honey, I realize you feel this is not a problem.

But I also feel it has a serious impact on our relationship. I love you and I don't want to feel resentment because I'm constantly repeating myself and interpreting for you. I find myself depressed and unable to figure out any better ways to cope with this. In life, you manage things better than most of us. Better than most people. But your hearing loss is a problem for us all. Our quality of life as a family would be so much better if you were willing to address this problem."

Therapist*:* "Tim, I think what we have to address is the upset in the lives of your family members as a result of your insistence on not wanting hearing aids. What if you actually hearing better also brought joy and tranquility to the rest of your family? What if Sue's depression was diminished by your efforts? Would you be willing to go the extra mile for them?"

There was a long silence. Nobody spoke. Tim got the message. The ultimate goal was for Tim to get hearing aids <u>for himself</u>, not others, but it took doing it for others before he realized the value it held for him. If his family didn't come together in a loving way, he may not have agreed to try hearing aids. He could have dug his heels in deeper and become even more defensive.

Some resistant hard-of-hearing people only need a nudge to get them to take action. Ideally, before the end of a family gathering, you want a commitment from your loved one that he will do something about his hearing problem, such as scheduling a hearing test, a screening or a hearing aid trial (most hearing healthcare practitioners offer at least 30-days). He must set a time, date and place for this action to occur and commit to seeing it through.

A Depression Screening

Some people are terribly affected by depression, something which holds them back from the joys life offers. At the time of this writing, there is a quick, free, 10-question online screening test for depression: www.med.nyu.edu/Psych/public.html.

If you go to this site, merely click on "The Online Depression Screening Test (ODST) (NYU)" to access it. New York University School of Medicine Department of Psychiatry sponsored it. This could turn out to be a very effective, private and safe way for you to inspire your loved one to assess his condition and seek help if depression is suspected.

You may want to check out Table 3-2 listing websites that may be of interest to you in the area of depression.

Treatment for Depression

Noteworthy in older adults is the prevalence of depression. Many elders spend time alone, not by choice. Their friends may have passed on, many are divorced or widowed, and the presence of hearing loss only drives them further into seclusion. If elders suffer from co-existing medical conditions, studies have shown that they are more likely to suffer the ramifications of depression.[15]

The most effective treatment for depression in older adults comes from medication, psychotherapy or a combination of both. In fact, research shows it is 80 percent effective.[16] The challenge with treatment is noncompliance—that is, patients who fail to take their prescribed medications or make the commitment to therapy.

It may be too great a challenge for an older person suffering from depression to address the issues of hearing loss without simultaneously

Table 3-2: Websites discussing depression (where applicable search keyword "depression").

www.apa.org
[American Psychological Association]

www.depression.org
[National Foundation for Depressive Illness]

www.med.nyu.edu
[New York University School of Medicine "Depression Screening"]

www.nami.org
[National Alliance for the Mentally Ill]

www.ndmda.org
[National Depressive and Manic Depressive Association]

www.nih.gov/nia
[National Institute on Aging]

www.nimh.nih.gov
[National Institute of Mental Health]

www.nmha.org
[National Mental Health Association]

www.nmisp.org
[National Mental Illness Screening Project]

www.psychwww.com/resource/journals.htm
[links to psychological journals]

treating the depressive disorder. Once in treatment, amplification would be better received and as a result of effective treatment, one's whole psychological perspective is likely to be more positive. Perhaps an ideal path to establish such treatment is your loved one's primary care physician who already holds a position of trust and guidance.

Fact: One study found that hard-of-hearing people who sought help through hearing aids experienced a 36 percent reduction in depression.[12]

Anxiety

Your loved one sits at the restaurant table smiling at a friend talking to the group. You can tell on his face that he's being polite as he struggles to understand each word. Your heart goes out to him, but there's really not much you can do. It's not a situation where you can interpret for him. Then he pops in with a statement that seems to come from left field. It makes no sense to anyone. A couple people even laugh, but he intended no humor in it. He suddenly realizes what he's done. You want to crawl under the table with him in embarrassment.

If your loved one suffers the consequences of hearing loss because he refuses assessment or treatment and he's already told you he hates the idea of wearing hearing aids, then this little story represents only a fraction of the situations both you and your loved one experience.

Anxiety is very commonly found among hard-of-hearing people. The experience of not hearing is associated with not feeling safe in conversations, misinterpreting words, responding inappropriately and feeling left out among people you love. These negative events can lead to frustrations, humiliations and embarrassments as well as anxiety. For some, it can lead to isolation that ends in despair.

Research Corroborates Hearing Loss with Anxiety

Research has now shown that as hearing loss progresses up to a moderate level, anxiety increases as well.[13] Moreover, if your loved one suffers from co-existing medical conditions including depression or alcoholism, there's an increased risk of anxiety.[17-19]

It's normal to experience anxieties if you are planning to make a public speech, take a test or meet with an employer who is assessing your work performance. Normal anxiety is typically associated with a particular stressor and is transient.

Adjustment Disorder with Anxiety

Anxiety disorders affect about 19,000,000 American adults.[20] They are serious medical illnesses which, if left untreated, grow worse. Probably the most common condition found among hard-of-hearing people is "Adjustment Disorder with Anxiety." *The Diagnostic and Statistical Manual of Mental Disorders*[21] states this is present when anxiety symptoms develop in response to an identifiable stressor that occurs within three months of the onset of the stressor (such as worsening hearing loss). Your loved one's symptoms could include feeling jittery, nervous, anxious or excessively worried. This distress would be greater than what would be expected from the loss of hearing alone.

In addition, these symptoms would carry over into your loved one's work and social functioning. Also, if one experiences anxiety, there is a high probability of the existence of depression. The bottom line is that coping abilities are taxed beyond what one can endure.

Among the phobias, "Specific Phobia" is commonly found among hard-of-hearing people. According to *The Diagnostic and Statistical Manual of Mental Disorders,*[21] this is a marked, persistent and excessive fear experienced in the presence of, or when anticipating an encounter with a specific object or situation that almost always provokes an immediate anxiety response. It would not be unusual for your loved one to recognize that the phobia is excessive or irrational. For example, if for six months or longer he avoids dinner engagements in restaurants because it causes him extreme anxiety, this is a specific phobia, despite the fact that he knows there is no real threat to him.

Table 3-3 shows other types of anxieties that might be exacerbated by hearing loss. If you can identify a type that corresponds to your loved one, you will want to explore this further with him and a therapist. One approach to ease into this discussion is to have him visit the same online site I recommended earlier for depression. Merely click on "The Online Screening for Anxiety (OSA) (NYU)" [www.med.nyu.edu/Psych/public.html]. At the time of this writing it is still available at no charge: It's a simple 10-question anxiety test.

Table 3-3: Other types of anxiety disorders may be exacerbated by hearing loss.[21-22]

[Note: to qualify as disorders, these conditions must result in at least 6 months of persistent and excessive anxiety and worry.]

Social phobia: persistent fear of social or performance situations in which embarrassment may occur. Example: avoidance of social gatherings for fear that hearing loss will cause embarrassment.

Post-traumatic stress disorder (PTSD): development of characteristic symptoms following exposure to an extreme traumatic stressor. Certain sounds often precipitate a startle reflex in sufferers, in turn triggering past trauma associations. Example: a veteran fitted with hearing aids hears the roar of a helicopter which now sounds abnormally loud, triggering an emotional response.

Generalized anxiety disorder: excessive anxiety and worry (occurring more days than not over at least 6 months) about a number of events or activities, and *not* due to a general medical condition.

Substance-induced anxiety disorder: prominent anxiety symptoms judged to be the direct physiological effects of a substance. Example: addiction to, and/or use of, alcohol or drugs can induce anxiety, which can render a person more susceptible to anxiety from other stressors, including poor hearing.

Treatment for Anxiety

Something not often considered is that the fear of not hearing (and choosing not to remedy the problem by hearing aid use) can itself become a process of progressive anxiety. Treatment for anxiety includes a program of psychotherapy and/or medication. When patients are compliant and stick to the program, the prognosis of a successful outcome is good. For more thorough treatment recommendations and exploration into anxiety, you might explore some of the websites listed below in Table 3-4 and/or consult your physician.

Table 3-4: Websites may be helpful in your search on anxiety. Many sites offer search capabilities.

---

www.adaa.org
[Anxiety Disorders Association of America]

www.freedomfromfear.com
[Freedom from Fear]

www.nami.org
[National Alliance for the Mentally Ill]

www.nimh.nih.gov
[National Institute of Mental Health]

www.nmha.org
[National Mental Health Association]

www.anxietynetwork.com
[The Anxiety Network International]

http://anxiety.psy.ohio-state.edu
[Ohio State University]

Emotions of the
Resistant Hard-of-Hearing Loved One

It should be mentioned that some hard-of-hearing people, depending on their temperament (and personality types of other family members) can live a relatively tranquil life with untreated hearing loss. These are people who believe they have a low demand for hearing and whose family has resigned themselves to the fact that their loved one not seeking treatment means living with this person the best way they can. It may not be an exemplary home life for communication, but one more of resignation, isolation and depression—especially among older married couples whose children are out of the house. This at best does not make life easy.

Key: Living with untreated hearing loss can be like living with a chronic disease—it never goes away and it usually gets worse.

If you want to capture a snapshot of the psychological characteristics that typically identify a resistant hard-of-hearing person as well as your own feelings about it, Table 3-5 delves deeply into this. Look at the list of recognized emotions commonly experienced by hard-of-hearing people, many even experienced by family members. You no doubt already realize the consequences of these emotions. Once again you must realize that you are not alone in your suffering through these conditions. Your own family and millions of others suffer with you.

Table 3-5: Common emotions experienced by hard-of-hearing people, many endured by the rest of the family are listed. Put a check on the left for those that pertain to him and a check on the right for those that pertain to you (for a better sense of how these emotions impact you and possibly the family).

__Ambivalence__	__Instability__
__Anger__	__Intolerances__
__Anxiety__	__Irritability__
__Arrogance__	__Isolation__
__Avoidance__	__Job Ineffectiveness__
__Confusion__	__Loneliness__
__Concentration__ (Difficulties)	__Negativism__
	__Nervousness__
__Defeat__	__Paranoia__
__Defensiveness__	__Phobias__
__Depression__	__Rejection__
__Discontentment__	__Resentment__
__Discouragement	__Safety Issues__
__Disorientation__	__Self-Criticism__
__Embarrassment__	__Self-Defeat__
__Fatigue__	__Self-Esteem Issues__
__Fear__	__Selfishness__
__Frustration__	__Shame__
__Hostility__	__Short-Tempered__
__Impatience__	__Stigmatized__
__Inadequacy__	__Stress__
__Inattentiveness__	__Temperamental__
__Incompetence__	__Tension__
__Inferiority__	__Upset Easily __
__Inflexibility__	__Vanity__
__Insecurity__	__Withdrawal__

> **Key: Examining the emotional character-**
> **istics of your loved one gives you**
> **insights on what needs to change.**

Despite the many descriptors you relate to in Table 3-5, the good news is that all these emotions and feelings caused by untreated hearing loss <u>can be reversed in many hard-of-hearing people</u> when the individual receives the benefits from hearing aids. Kochkin and Rogin[13] reported precisely these findings. They found the top three areas of improvements for both the hard-of-hearing person and family members included:

- *relationships at home*
- *feelings about oneself*
- *life overall*

These are impressive findings! They should encourage you not to give up your quest to help your loved one. Now that you have insight on these emotions, you need to determine what to do about them. The best way to address them is to share these feelings with your loved one. He needs to know how his hearing loss impacts you. This must be achieved through loving discussion, not through accusations and intimidations. This list can also be a great tool for opening discussion with a therapist. If your loved one is also willing to complete the list, it will give the therapist insights into the conflicts between you both.

To better understand the dynamics of untreated hearing loss, you only need to look at how the world closes in on such an individual (discussed next).

Auditory Desensitization

In a "sixth sense" sort of way, we can almost hear with our eyes and see with our ears. Think about it. When someone talks to you from another room, you can't see them, but you can often hear and understand them if you have normal hearing and they're not too far away. Sometimes you can even sense where in the room they're sitting. In this way, you are "seeing" around a corner by hearing them. These sounds are reassuring and add to our sense of safety. For example, if a child is playing in another room, often all it takes is hearing him play to know he's safe.

The first things that hard-of-hearing people lose are the sounds that orient them. Common sounds to which you pay no attention—like the refrigerator motor, heating or cooling through air ducts, the tick of a clock, footsteps, water running, ice stirred in a glass, the sound of the computer or printer running—orient you in your environment. While you may even consider these sounds at times annoying, they are in fact essential to your orientation and security. Their absence would be greatly missed, as you can experience by inserting earplugs in your ears. What results for hard-of-hearing people is a closing in of their world.

When these sounds are only faintly audible or disappear altogether, which can occur with mild high frequency hearing loss, the world in which one lives and the reality to which one responds exists within a shorter distance around them (depending on the severity of the loss). What can result is *auditory desensitization to sounds*. That is, for example, sounds that cannot be correctly processed and identified yet nevertheless are "heard" (like a fork heard dropping onto a plate from another room but unidentified) are simply ignored. The brain does not know what to do with this information. To the brain, it's abstract information, so it learns to ignore it.

This eventually occurs for speech sounds as well. You call to your loved one from across the room but he does not respond. What he hears is meaningless speech sounds, like a fork dropping on a plate. The brain doesn't process it as meaningful information. He hears you speak but doesn't get that you are speaking to him. The words are recognized as speech, but not understood.

Understand that while we receive sound in our ears, we actually "hear" with our brains. Sounds are given meaning in the brain by reflecting pictures in your mind. These interpreted pictures do not exist if you do not hear the corresponding sounds. The collection of these "pictures" you do hear comprises a meaningful portion of your reality. Therefore, what you hear and what you do not hear shapes behavior and attitudes.

Among those with untreated hearing loss, when this auditory desensitization progresses far enough with reduced auditory stimulation (such as a person with loss of hearing in both ears but wears only one hearing aid), *late onset auditory deprivation* can result in the unaided ear—a more rapid decline in speech recognition due to inadequate stimulation of cochlear structures.[23-24]

Early in the process of losing some hearing, a person may make inquiry into what the sound was, but this behavior (of trying to make meaning out of meaningless sound) is usually extinguished over time because one realizes it was a "normal sound" that one simply could not fully process. As a result, another behavior kicks in—that of learning to ignore sounds that do not make sense. This becomes a learned behavior purely a result of how the mind automatically purges useless information it "hears." You do this all the time. You ignore a computer hum, crickets chirping, people chatting in another room. The only difference with hearing loss is that this process is not voluntary. It's out of their control. While you can "tune it out," much of the sound in their world is already tuned out.

Sounds that are not tuned out by hard-of-hearing people, but are partially audible, may result in a startle if it cannot be identified. This is especially problematic among older people. Have you ever been alone at night and heard a sound that you couldn't identify? Did it scare you? In more vulnerable (and typically older) people, it can make their environment feel terribly unsafe and even begin to conjure up feelings of paranoia.

The bad news is the downward spiral of this cycle. The longer one goes being unable to identify sounds one should hear, the more the brain becomes either confused or learns to ignore these signals. In a situation that already poses problems because of hearing loss, we now add to this further deterioration a lack of stimulation of the hair cells of the inner ear. This auditory deprivation may lead to permanent damage to the auditory receiving and regulatory centers of the brain that interpret sound.

Suddenly, something as innocent as just not wanting to get hearing aids becomes a health crisis in the auditory system. It also imposes changes in one's personal communication and lifestyle and directly affects the entire family's quality of life.

The use of hearing aids early enough after auditory deprivation has occurred <u>can result in improved speech understanding in the aided ear</u>. However, when two hearing aids are indicated but only one is worn, there remains that risk of progressive reduction in speech recognition in the unaided ear.

Chapter 4

Solutions

Chapter 4

Solutions

In Chapter 2 we established 10 steps to your loved one's *independent hearing*. Now let's explore a solid foundation on which these steps can rest. There are *three easy steps* you can take to achieve the success you are looking for. I will discuss each of them, but you must decide how they apply in your specific situation.

1. Recognize Life Patterns in You Both

We are all creatures of habit. Not only does your loved one have fairly predictable habits, but you do too. You both typically get up at a certain time, eat at a certain time, watch specific television shows on favorite nights, make long distance phone calls to the kids on certain days and so forth. You may not do these together, but the timeline is often predictable. Similarly, the way in which your loved one manages his health and associated problems is predictable. He may be fanatical or ambivalent. He may be someone who enjoys talking about it but doing nothing, or someone who can't even discuss his hearing problem. These patterns are established early in life by our personalities—the kind of person we are. Recognizing his patterns of behavior and attitude will give you the information you need to know how to work with him in order to surmount them.

If your loved one is hesitant to discuss his own hearing problem, then you must discuss with him the effects of his condition on you, the kids, loved ones and friends. In this quest, you cannot use angry words to describe his failure to address the problem. You must merely enlighten him to how much more difficult life is for you and others because of his lack of treatment.

Sixty-eight year old Mary does this effectively: "Honey, I need to tell you, this is very hard for me. Having to repeat things constantly is exhausting by the end of the day. I cannot raise my voice anymore to have you hear like you need to. I love you very much but you need to understand my own limitations."

Mary underwent by-pass surgery years earlier and lost much of the power in her voice. She is unable to project her voice like she had prior to surgery, but this doesn't mean her husband has stopped expecting her to talk louder. Many men and women over age seventy have reduced capability to project their voices.

Part of this pattern you'll need to explore is your own role. Have you been assisting him for so long that he now expects it? If so, you are part of his pattern. This is one of the co-dependency issues discussed earlier. It is now time for you to change your pattern if you expect to help him. You need to lovingly tell him you'll no longer repeat yourself and then make a conscious effort not to interpret for him.

2. Identify the Challenges

If you recognize the patterns of your loved one, then you also know the challenges that face you. He tells you ambivalently, "I know I don't hear like I used to, but I'm not going to wear one of those things in my ear!"

Make him clear about *your challenge*. From the earlier intervention with Sue and Tim, here's more of Sue's reasoning:

"I know you don't want to wear hearing aids. However, I'm no longer willing to interpret for you when we're out with our friends. Many of them have voiced their concern to me about you. Just last week, Ruth asked me if you might have had a stroke because you weren't able to correctly write down the directions she was dictating to you."

Another option for your resistant hard-of-hearing loved one is to videotape him in a situation where he struggles. A family celebration may be a perfect opportunity to do this in a non-threatening way. Engage him in conversation even though you know it will be challenging, so you can document the experience. Engage others at the same time, assuming that they can hear you.

In order to avoid any risk of embarrassment, later in private, replay the video for your loved one. It should be readily apparent to him that everyone else was capable of conversing and he wasn't. This can be a very enlightening moment. You may not need to do anything other than just play the video. Sometimes, like they say, a picture is worth a thousand words. Give him the opportunity to mull this over in his mind.

If eventually this does not bring you the results you're after, you can repeat it in another environment (ideally even at home in the living room if he has difficulty there).

3. Commit to the Changes

Commit to no longer being an enabler by not repeating and interpreting. Once you make your mind up that you will not settle for anything less than what is best for your loved one, you can make it happen. You cannot force it, but you can create it. No one likes being pushed, but when gentle, helpful guidance in the form of love and compassion comes, miracles can happen.

Here's an example of daughter Bonnie who committed to changing her enabling behavior with her father, who was continually asking the family to repeat a part of their storytelling. "Dad, we would really like you to be part of the conversation, but in order to do that, you will have to deal with your hearing loss because none of us are willing to continue with the frustrations of repeating ourselves." Don't be afraid to be tough but loving. Your tone of voice is as important as what you say.

Confronting Excuses

Before your loved one can think about treatment, look at what resistant hard-of-hearing people report as their rationales for not getting help. Table 4-1 shows what 2,304 hard-of-hearing respondents ages 50 and older reported.

Addressing Resistance (Denial)

In Table 4-1 under Denial, if your loved one feels his *"Hearing isn't bad enough"* or he *"Can get along without hearing aids,"* then obviously he feels it isn't as bad as you or others believe it to be. The fact that he knows he has some hearing loss actually disqualifies it as being denial, so the term is used more figuratively.

Readily apparent is that more than two-thirds of respondents felt their hearing loss was *"Not bad enough yet to get help."* You may ask how they

Table 4-1: Reasons resistant hard-of-hearing people give for not using hearing aids.

Denial -	Everyone in Study	Those with Milder Loss	Those with Severe Loss
My hearing isn't bad enough	69%	73%	64%
I can get along without one.	68%	78%	55%
Consumer Concerns –			
Too expensive.	55%	48%	64%
Won't help my specific problem.	33%	31%	36%
I heard they don't work well.	28%	26%	31%
I don't trust hearing specialists.	25%	22%	29%
I tried one and it didn't work.	17%	15%	20%
Stigma and Vanity –			
Makes me feel old.	20%	18%	22%
I don't like the way they look.	19%	18%	21%
I'm too embarrassed to wear one.	18%	16%	21%
Don't like what others will think about me.	16%	15%	19%

Reprinted from The National Council on the Aging, Seniors Research Group and Market Strategies Inc., 1999, 409 Third St. SW, Suite 200, Washington, DC 20024.

could think such a thing when they cannot hear! Most of their interpretation was based on misinformation. This held true for people even in the severe hearing loss category (where unaided, they would not hear a telephone or doorbell ring or any meaningful conversation across a table). It makes you wonder just how bad must it get before one would feel help was necessary?

As stated emphatically over and over in this book, you must stop being his ears: stop repeating, stop interpreting and give him the chance from his own experience to learn just how bad his condition really is without you compensating for what he cannot hear.

Without making your loved one wrong or having him feel bad about his problem, without falling back into co-dependency, you must confront his fallacious defenses with insightful and intelligent responses about the problem that will inspire change (presented next).

Addressing Consumer Concerns

With respect to "Consumer Concerns" in Table 4-1, foremost is a cost-benefit issue for more than half of those surveyed, suggesting that *"Hearing aids are too expensive."* This is based largely on myths and rumors. Hard-of-hearing people tend to believe that the expense of hearing aids may not result in a proportional value for the dollars spent. This is untrue.

The value of certain style hearing aids has been assessed in two reports[25-26] compared with other industries, reported by The American Customer Satisfaction Index (ACSI).[27] The ACSI annually reports measures of quality and performance for many products and services by percentile ranking. Such staunch standbys in 2002 were reported for health insurance companies (satisfaction rating of 68%), broadcast TV (satisfaction rating of 65%), newspapers (satisfaction rating of 63%), fast food restaurants (satisfaction rating of 62%) and even the Food and Drug Administration (satisfaction rating of 68%)—what's more reliable than the government testing our food and drugs? I'll tell you what ranked higher: programmable hearing aids with directional microphones (satisfaction rating of 81-82%, respectively).[25-26]

This demonstrates that the flexibility in programming significantly increases the chances for satisfaction with hearing aids when consumers can spend the extra money (for programmability). Thus, it should not be surprising when we see research confirm our suspicions that: "...*benefit* when compared to *price* overwhelmingly explains the majority of customer satisfaction...[and] indicates that consumers on average are perhaps more forgiving on price when benefit is high."[25]

Here are some examples of questions you can ask in response to your loved one's issues:

He says: *They are too expensive.*
Ideas for response:

- "How much are they?"
- "Who quoted the price?"
- "What did the quote include? Digital? Multiple microphones? Multiple programs?"
- "Price is relative—what's it worth for you to hear better?"
- "Did you read that one study showed 76 percent of people who own hearing aids are satisfied with their benefit?"[28]

He says: *Won't help my specific problem.*
Ideas for response:

- "What is your specific problem?" (Get him to identify it.)
- "How do you know this problem cannot be helped?" (Did a hearing healthcare practitioner say so?)
- "Are you willing to take a 30-day trial to prove it one way or the other to us both?"

He says: *I heard they don't work well.*
Ideas for response:

- "What is your source of information?" (Rumors are unreliable. One person's bad experience cannot justify another person's lack of action.)
- "Have you tried them yourself for your specific problem?"
- "Have you read the latest literature and research?"

He says: *I don't trust hearing specialists.*
Ideas for response:

- "Do you have firsthand experience?"
- "How many have you visited?"
- "Isn't it in your best hearing healthcare interests to consider seeing somebody?"

He says: *I tried one and it didn't work.*
Ideas for response (assuming he actually tried one):

- "How long ago was that and do you think technology has changed since then?"
- "Have you considered consulting with someone else?"

Stigma and Vanity

The world in which we live venerates good looks, classy dress, peak sexual performance, the perfect diet, the best workout program, exuberant personalities, radiant health, and that we should all be living a more "Hollywood" lifestyle. Daytime and evening television commercials support these illusions regarding how we ought to live our lives. If you turn on television in the wee hours of the morning, you cannot miss seeing one infomercial after another touting promise for better living.

These kinds of repeated bombardments in advertising can make healthy and psychologically sound people feel guilty and inadequate. If one suffers from a handicap or disability, it can make them feel even worse. The idea portrayed is that we should look our best and give the impression of ideal health. However, this just is not reality.

Most of us think of vanity as a condition to simply "get over," but vanity can run to the core of a person's spirit, directing their lives. Research shows that many people who experience vanity feel worthless and empty inside.

The impact of these kinds of messages from television, radio, newsprint and now the Internet is not always healthy. A hard-of-hearing person who feels terrible about having lost some hearing may not be ready to acknowledge this problem. The message they get from this media onslaught is that they better look their best. Folding back one deeper layer of the onion finds them assuming that wearing hearing aids will prevent them from looking their best. Hence, they feel stigmatized rather than realizing hearing aids are actually their solution—amplification enhances and improves both communication skills and self-image.

Yet, vanity issues continue to hold back many potential hearing aid candidates from benefiting, either because they have not made that first step of trying them or they tried them and failed on the first go-around. Some are stuck in between. They purchase the smallest hearing aids available that are cosmetically attractive, but they require more power than can be packed into that little space. Thus, they look great, but they still can't hear!

This is a tragic commentary on the social stigma placed on wearing hearing aids by some people. It has its basis in fear (of what others might think). This group of hard-of-hearing people would prefer to face the humiliations, embarrassments and frustrations of not hearing (or hearing poorly with the wrong hearing aids) in order to present themselves to the world as "whole," "perfect" and "well."

The truth is they perceive themselves as lacking something for which they need to cover up. They may have fragile egos. Their self-esteem may be low. Just as unfortunate, they expect you to compensate for what they feel they are lacking. The closer you are to this loved one, the greater the conflict often becomes, especially if you're married to this problem because there seems to be no escape.

His vanity may not stop at hearing aids. It can extend to anything that could cause him to feel stigmatized: loss of hair, obesity, some kind of disfigurement, skin conditions and so forth. Resistance to hearing aids merely brings out the behavior inherently a part of who he already is.

A scenario relayed to me by a patient's loved one represents a common vanity issue. Gladys, Phillip and their two grown children were out to dinner in a restaurant with moderate noise (average for an open dining area seating 75 people). Very soft, live music by one synthesizer player added to the drone. Everyone exchanged loving thoughts except Phillip who sat glumly at the table hardly uttering a word. The family knew he didn't hear because he wouldn't get hearing aids, but they also knew they could not continually repeat and interpret conversation after conversation since it was just not practical.

As the others observed Phillip it appeared he didn't care. He seemed absorbed with his filet mignon and baked potato and very happy to spend his dinnertime looking at his food rather than family members, though he occasionally glanced up and smiled at one of the family, or nodded agreeably.

When this story was relayed to me, the children perceived it as dad just being more engrossed in his dinner than with them (fully recognizing he could not hear well in the restaurant). They felt the hearing loss really did not bother him. But consider this. Do you think this situation of watching others interact and not hearing brought much pleasure to Phillip? For him, it was kind of like watching a silent film.

This is the illusion with vanity and stigma. Phillip seemed to make the best of his unfortunate circumstances by giving the illusion of contentment. The truth is he felt terrible, but he couldn't express it. I know this because only months after I fit him successfully with hearing aids he told me how he felt. What eventually drove him to see me was his absolute sense of isolation, something he could not express to his own family.

Phillip's case represents what I mentioned earlier about the world closing in on a hard-of-hearing person who does not seek help. At the dinner table in the restaurant, Phillip could not hear well enough to engage in intelligent conversation. Thus, his world shrunk literally to about a foot around him, comprising the only meaningful thing to which he could relate—his food. He could not even hear his son beside him well enough to understand what he said.

Phillip was not content. He was, however, more willing to put up with these kinds of indignities for years rather than confront the truth of his hearing problem and do something about it. He developed sophisticated avoidances. His behavior entailed limiting conversation to the quiet of his home. In the car, he would sing or listen to his music to avoid conversation. If shopping with his wife meant being around even mild noise, he'd pull a book or news-paper from beneath his arm and proceed to sit and read. Not because he was an avid reader, but because he was drawn to it by his avoidance behav-iors.

Avoidance of meaningful social gatherings can result in concomitant increases in paranoia, anxiety, depression, or for that matter, any of the symptoms cited in Table 3-5. <u>Hearing loss is no small matter</u>. It holds profound social and emotional conse-quences that can completely alter the way in which a person would like to live. In the prcoess it damages the closest relationships in life year after year until treatment.

Disconcerting under "Stigma/Vanity" (in Table 4-1) among those in the study is that it took the degree of hearing loss to worsen <u>before they would seek treatment</u>. This does not happen among eyeglasses wearers. As soon as we don't see well, we get glasses. And it certainly doesn't happen with common diseases. Then why should it happen among hearing aid candidates who, devoid of any direct experience with hearing aids, falsely conclude the devices will not work for them?

The basis for resistance will vary from person to person and can be much like peeling away layers of that onion. Once the layers of emotions are revealed and the core of resistance is exposed, you will discover it is often based in either *fear* or *shame*.

Key: Feelings of fear over what hearing aids cannot do are almost always based on what he does not know and held in place by a single bad event, myths, false assumptions or readily believable but untrue rumors.

This fear surrounds one's own misconceived notions of how hearing aids will impact one's life. Again, you get an idea of what it feels like in Table 4-1 under "Stigma/Vanity:" *It will make me look too old; I don't like the way they look; I'm too embarrassed; I don't like what others will think about me.*

Now read these again and imagine these same fears coming from a child expressing concern over wearing a particular article of clothing to school. You may chuckle, but it's the same fear whether expressed by a child or an adult, and the issue itself might seem to you to be absurd, but to your loved one, it is a profound, life-altering concern. These concerns must be respected and addressed.

At the core of the onion you may also find shame. While we may think of shame more closely associated with hiding a mental disorder, substance or sexual abuse, hearing loss can make some people feel ashamed. That is, they feel foolish or humiliated over what they do not hear or ashamed over their poor communication skills due to hearing loss. It has its basis in truth from their own experience. One self-defeating downside to shame is that it leads to low self-esteem.

For some, these feelings can dissolve as quickly as the time it takes to put hearing aids in the ears. For others, the hearing aid intensifies these ill feelings. It's all about one's readiness for help.

If you have issues with your loved one about stigma and vanity, here are some responses for you to consider:

He says: *It would make me feel old.*
Ideas for response:

- "How old do you feel when people mistakenly think you have cognitive issues instead of a hearing problem?"
- "Would you rather people think that something is more seriously wrong with you than your hearing?"

He says: *I don't like the way they look.*
Ideas for response:

- "Do you know how you look to others when you continually don't hear?"
- "Do you know what hearing aids look like nowadays?"
- "When was the last time you explored this question with a hearing healthcare practitioner?"

He says: *I'm too embarrassed to wear one.*
Ideas for response:

- "What is more embarrassing, suffering with not hearing or wearing hearing aids?"
- "A hearing loss is more noticeable than a hearing aid."

He says: *I don't like what <u>others</u> will think about me.*
Ideas for response:

- "Why is what others think more important than what's in your best interest?"
- "Your family also happens to be part of those <u>others</u> you refer to, and we think your quality of life is important enough for you to get help."

Key: Don't wait until he gets a handle on stigma and vanity before he gets hearing aids. Wearing hearing aids is the fastest way to conquer vanity.

The resistant hard-of-hearing spouse can be so absorbed in his own dilemma that he fails to recognize his hearing problems impact you in any meaningful way. In a selfish sort of the world-revolves-around-him attitude, he may on one hand appreciate the help you offer him in filling in gaps and repeating, but he does not see the hardship it imposes on you. He doesn't because he is not in touch with the reality of his problem. If he was in touch with the hardship his problem imposed on you, he may be more inclined to do something about it because he loves you.

Key: If you are to solve his hearing problems as they relate to you, influence a change in his thinking.

Hence, it is essential that you speak to him about the hardships his problem imposes on you. He must know this in order to change and ultimately seek treatment. He must also confront the fact that he is not fooling anyone. He needs to understand how he can appear foolish or senile, disinterested in or rude to people he loves when he does not realize someone is talking to him; or seemingly dazed or cognitively impaired, such as recovering from a stroke. Resistant hard-of-hearing people rarely get to see this slice of reality on themselves because people are too uncomfortable or polite to say anything to them about their hearing loss.

You must not make him "look good" and cover for his communication errors. If you believe your loved one is vain, let the vanity run its course. Allow him to fumble so he can grasp the depth of his problem. I know this sounds cruel, but devoid of other alternatives, these unfortunate consequences are one clear path to his enlightenment and long-term healing.

Sadly, what most resistant hard-of-hearing people seldom realize is what you see—your perspective—his true persona when he does not hear. If he was able to see through your eyes and others, the basis for his resistance would crumble.

See a Hearing Health Care Practitioner

If he will not consult with a hearing healthcare practitioner, then you go alone. Meet the hearing healthcare practitioner. While literature is often helpful to those who are ready for treatment, too much can be overwhelming. Would he respond more favorably to reading one brochure you could take home with you from the hearing healthcare practitioner's office? Might a book be a better solution? You know best how much is too much.

Ask the hearing healthcare practitioner if he or she offers free seminars in the community to which you and your loved one could attend without obligation. Hearing healthcare practitioners often hold open houses a few times a year. This could be another option for you both. Find out times and dates. These kinds of informal and very relaxed gatherings are ideal and safe environments for your loved one.

If your hearing healthcare practitioner's office offers *aural rehabilitation classes*, you have found a perfect resource. These classes offer education, guidance and counseling to new hearing aid wearers. It's an opportunity for your loved one to become acquainted with other people experiencing similar problems and see firsthand how others are benefiting from hearing aids. You both will meet others with the same problems you have. You personally will meet other family members enduring the identical frustrations and agonies you live through daily. You will hear from others about the painful challenges that took years to surmount. Here's another opportunity to discover you're not alone.

Sometimes you both can attend a session as guests even if your loved one has not gone through a hearing assessment yet. However, having the hearing exam first will assist the hearing healthcare practitioner in better addressing specific issues your loved one may have. If he declines the assessment but will go to one class, you are still light years ahead in doing so. These classes are invaluable, though unfortunately, only a minority of hearing healthcare practitioners provide them. (They are time-consuming for busy practitioners.)

Facts: When you consider the numbers, it can seem disheartening. According to the National Institute on Deafness and Other Communication Disorders (NIDCD):[29]

- **About 30-35 percent of the U.S. population between the ages of 65 and 75 years have a hearing loss.**

- **It is estimated that 40-50 percent of people 75 and older have a hearing loss.**

- **In 1989, the NIDCD reported that hearing loss was the third most prevalent chronic condition affecting older Americans.**

Research backs logical deduction that when spouses, family members, loved ones and friends take an active role in the hearing rehabilitation process, the hard-of-hearing person responds more favorably to treatment, progresses faster in adjustment to hearing aids and he develops higher self-esteem. As a matter of fact, it's worth reviewing Table 3-5. All these conditions are reversible and your loved one will be more apt to resolve them when you offer vigilant support. This does not mean repeating yourself constantly. It means directing him in ways that will resolve his dependency on you and others and ultimately lead to his *hearing independence* and resolution of his hearing problem.

Key: If you do nothing, the odds are about five-to-one against your loved one taking action.

Hearing Aid Selection

Once you find a way to encourage and inspire your loved one to seek the needed help, you need to be willing to get involved. This means accompanying your loved one to the hearing healthcare practitioner's office, listening to what is involved in the process of hearing aids <u>and being willing to be an integral part of his process toward better hearing</u>. *This is not co-dependency.* This is loving and nurturing support so long as he takes the lead.

Key: You should support your loved one by accompanying him on every visit to the hearing healthcare practitioner's office within the first 30-60 days.

You may have to take instruction on how hearing aids work; how they're inserted in the ears; how to recognize when batteries are dead and how to replace them; how to keep hearing aids clean; and assist him as needed. If the hearing healthcare practitioner and your loved one welcome the idea, you may include another family member or friend. Often, the greater the support, the better he will feel about his experience.

The goal here is assistance. It is nobody else's role to perform his hearing aid responsibilities unless there are problems that prevent him from doing them (for example, arthritis so severe he cannot change hearing aid batteries, or memory problems that prevent recall of hearing aid functions, etc.). There may be a lot of information to retain once he gets hearing aids. Provide whatever necessary help that will lead toward his independence.

Some people require up to several months to be comfortable enough to go it alone. He may not be able to express it to you, but your support will mean the world to him.

Once you get your loved one into the hearing healthcare practitioner's office for the initial assessment, he may give you another set of challenges including the type and style of hearing aids <u>he</u> wants—rather than what will best serve his needs (according to what the hearing healthcare practitioner recommends). He may want an "invisible" set of hearing aids. He may want the least expensive. He may want the style he sees your neighbor wearing or the kind he read about in a magazine ad. The hearing aid selection process must be a mutually agreed on determination. However, if the hearing healthcare practitioner feels your loved one's particular selection would compromise hearing ability, this is the wrong choice. When competently fitted, hearing aids transform lives.

If you are consulting with a hearing healthcare practitioner, you will be guided to wipe the slate clean of preconceived ideas of what is best for him. In an ideal world, it should be the hearing healthcare practitioner recommending what your loved one should be using. Naturally, cost is a factor. But if you offer a budget, your hearing healthcare practitioner can work within it.

For example, 100 percent digital hearing aids

used to be a lot pricier. These hearing aids are now manufactured across a broad spectrum of costs and options and are affordable to more people than ever before.

Receiving treatment does not only mean your loved one is getting on his feet. It will positively affect the entire family. Kochkin and Rogin[13] reported dramatic improvements for the entire family following treatment. Look at the impact you and your loved one can expect:

- Reduction in anger and frustration
- Reduction in anxiety, social phobias, depression and depressive symptoms
- Reduction in feelings of paranoia
- Reduction in discrimination toward the person with the hearing loss
- Reduction in difficulty associated with communication (primarily severe to profound hearing losses)
- Reduction in compensatory behaviors and idiosyncrasies
- Reduced self-criticism
- Improved sense of control in your life
- Improved cognitive functioning (primarily severe to profound hearing loss)
- Improved interpersonal relationships (especially for mild-moderate losses) including greater intimacy and lessening of negative dysfunctional communication
- Improved health status and less incidence of pain
- Enhanced emotional stability
- Enhanced group social activity
- Greater earning power (especially in severe hearing losses)

Dr. Kochkin reports that the evidence is compelling: "In this study, both respondents and their family members were asked to independently rate the extent to which they believed their life was specifically improved due to hearing aids. All hearing loss groups from mild to profound reported significant improvements in nearly every area measured:

- Relationships at home and with family
- Feelings about self
- Life overall
- Mental health
- Social life
- Emotional health
- Physical health

"I believe this study challenges every segment of society to comprehend the devastating impact of hearing loss on individuals and their families as well as the positive possibilities associated with hearing aid usage."[2] (Pages 74; 76)

Fact: The only factor with more influence than you in driving a loved one's decision to pursue hearing aids is the hearing loss getting worse.[30]

It's worth mentioning that if you or your loved one depend on your physician for guidance, you would be well-advised to know that research reveals only 14 percent of physicians screen for hearing loss[31] and many of them perceive that hearing loss in the older population is merely *an inevitable process of aging with nothing to be done.* (This does not include medical specialists in hearing such as otologists or otolaryngologists who are well-read and keenly aware of these problems.) Therefore, if you are so advised by a well-meaning physician, you need to know that this is not helpful advice.

Take a Moment to Listen

One of the most important things you can do as a loving spouse, friend or family member is *listen*. Listening is an art and often difficult for people. Once you are able to inspire your loved one to face his resistance, you need to listen to how he feels about it. You need to give him the space to express his fears, shame and concerns to you. Remember, this is a big breakthrough for many resistant hard-of-hearing people. If you were successful in planting the seeds of inspiration that will hopefully lead him to action, let him now take the lead. Encourage open dialogue while being careful of coercion.

Earlier in this book you were faced with your hard-of-hearing loved one implying, "If you love me, you'll help me (hear)." Now that you have a better understanding of the complexities of your relationship with him, you can recognize that the solution to resolving your crisis is *you saying to him,* "If you love me, you'll get help," a less co-dependent response.

If you express to your loved one how deeply you love him, how sincerely you want what's best for him, it is the most direct and profound communication you can offer. I truly believe that despite how elementary it sounds, the expression of love can move mountains. If you look again at the emotions listed in Table 3-5 (on page 68), you will quickly observe that they all are obstacles to healthy relationships and expressions of love. If you can make the effort to surmount them, this is the basis on which all future communication with your loved one depends.

Final Thoughts

At the beginning I stated that figuring out how to approach your loved one would require a quiet mind, a resilient spirit, compassion, willpower, patience, well-defined goals that follow an organized plan, knowledge of hearing healthcare in your community and ultimately willingness to change on your part and on the part of your loved one.

My greatest hope for you is attainment of these possibilities. And they are attainable. If you follow the guidelines and suggestions in this book, you can't fail to positively impact your loved one. Stop being his ears, begin discussing the issues, consider all options and offer your loving support. In doing so, you can expect not only improvements in his hearing and communication once he's treated, but a higher quality of life for the entire family.

While this is the end of the book, I hope it's just the beginning of a richly rewarding journey for you and your loved one. I wish you every success.

References

1. Carmen R. Who is more resistant to hearing aid purchases – women or men? *Audiology Today*, 2005; 17 (2): in press.

2. Carmen R. (Ed.) *The Consumer Handbook on Hearing Loss & Hearing Aids: A Bridge to Healing* (Second Edition). Sedona: Auricle Ink Publishers, 2004.

3. *New Oxford American Dictionary.* New York: Oxford University Press, 2001.

4. In NIH publication No. 99-4584: Narrow WE. One-year prevalence of depressive disorders among adults 18 and over in the U.S.: NIMH ECA prospective data. Population estimates based on the US census estimated residential population age 18 and over on July 1, 1998: unpublished.

5. Murray CJL, Lopez AD, eds. *The Global Burden of Disease and Injury Series, Volume 1: A Comprehensive Assessment of Mortality and Disability from Diseases, Injuries, and Risk Factors in 1990 and Projected to 2020*. Cambridge, MA: Harvard University Press (Harvard School of Public Health on behalf of the World Health Organization and the World Bank), 1996.

6. Reiger DA, Narrow WE, Rae DS, et al. The de facto mental and addictive disorders service system. Epidemiologic Catchment Area prospective 1-year prevalence rates of disorders and services. *Archives of General Psychiatry*, 1993; 50 (2): 85-94.

7. Bridges JA, Bentler RA. Relating hearing aid use to well-being among older adults. *The Hearing Journal* 1998; 51 (7): 39-44.

8. Wallhagen MI, Strawbridge WJ, Kaplan GA. Six-year impact of hearing impairment on psychosocial and physiologic functioning. *Nurse Pract* 1996; 21 (9): 11-12; 14.

9. Strawbridge WJ, Wallhagen MI, Shema SJ, et al. Negative consequences of hearing impairment in old age: a longitudinal analysis. *The Gerontologist* 2000; 40 (3): 320-326.

10.www.nimh.nih.gov/publicat/elderlydepsuicide.cf m, NIH Publication No. 01-4593, 2001.

11. *Patient Care Advisor*, LRP Publications, 747 Dresher Rd., PO Box 980, Horsham PA 19044-0980, 1998.

12. www.ncoa.org.

13. Kochkin S and Rogin CM. Quantifying the obvious: the impact of hearing instruments on quality of life. *The Hearing Review* 2000; 7 (1): 8-34.

14. DiMatteo MR, Lepper HS, Croghan TW. Depression is a risk factor for noncompliance with medical treatment. *Arch Intern Med* 2000; 160 (14): 2101-07.

15. Schultz R, Beach SR, Ives DG, et al. Association between depression and mortality in older adults. *Arch Intern Med* 2000; 160 (12): 1761-68.

16. Little JT, Reynolds CF III, Dew MA, et al. How common is resistance to treatment in recurrent, nonpsychotic geriatric depression? *Amer J of Psychiatry* 1998; 155 (8): 1035-8.

17. Kendler KS, Neale MC, Kessler RC, et al.: Major depression and generalized anxiety disorder. Same genes, (partly) different environment? *Arch Gen Psychiat* 1992; 49: 716-722.

18. Reiger DA, Rae DS, Narrow WE, et al.: Prevalence of anxiety disorders and their comor-bidity with mood and addictive disorders. *Brit J*

Psychiat Suppl. 1998; 34: 24-28.

19. Agoub M, Asmaa E: Comorbidity of anxiety and depressive disorders in a primary care setting. Abstract CL-31.A. In *Program and Abstracts from World Psychiatric Association International Jubilee Congress*. Paris, France: June, 2000.

20. National Institute of Mental Health: *Anxiety Disorders*. NIH Publication No. 00-3879. Rockville, MD: NIMH, 1994.

21. American Psychiatric Association: *Diagnostic and Statistical Manual of Mental Disorders*, fourth ed., text revision. Washington, DC: American Psychiatric Association, 2000.

22. Carmen R. Hearing loss and anxiety in adults. *The Hearing Journal* 2002; 55 (4): 48-54.

23. Silman S, et al. Late onset auditory deprivation: effects of monaural versus binaural hearing aids. *J. Acoust. Soc. Am.* 1984; 76: 1357-62.

24. Silman S, et al. Adult onset auditory deprivation. *J. Am. Acad. Audiol* 1992; 3: 390-96.

25. Kochkin S. On the issue of value: hearing aid benefit, price, satisfaction and brand repurchase rates. *The Hearing Review* 2003; 10 (2): 12-25.

26. Schuchman G, Valente M, Beck LB and Potts MS. User satisfaction with an ITE directional hearing instrument. *The Hearing Review* 1999; 6 (7): 12; 16; 21-22.

27. The American Customer Satisfaction Index: http://www.theacsi.org, 2004.

28. Kochkin S. Ten-year customer satisfaction trends in the U.S. hearing instrument market. *The Hearing Review* 2002; 9 (10): 14-25; 46.

29. National Institute on Deafness and Other Communication Disorders: http://www.nidcd.nih

.gov/health/hearing/presbycusis.asp, 2004.

30. Kochkin S. MarketTrak IV: correlates of hearing aid purchase intent. *The Hearing Journal* 1998; 51 (1): 30-41.

31. Kochkin S. MarkeTrak VI. *The Hearing Review* 2001; 8 (12): 16-24.

INDEX

H